NEUROLOGY

MANAGEMENT OF COMMON DISEASES IN FAMILY PRACTICE

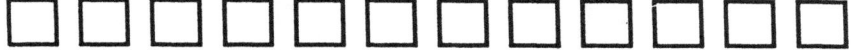

Series Editors: J. Fry and M. Lancaster-Smith

NEUROLOGY

T. J. Fowler, DM, FRCP

*Consultant Neurologist to the Dartford,
Greenwich and Tunbridge Wells Health Districts*

and

R. W. May, MB, BS, MRCGP

Principal in General Practice, Chislehurst, Kent

Springer-Science+Business Media, B.V.

British Library Cataloguing in Publication Data

Fowler, T.
  Neurology – (Management of common diseases
  in family practice)
  1. Nervous system – Diseases
  I. Title   II. May, R.W.   III. Series
  616.8   RC 346

  ISBN 978-94-010-9546-4   ISBN 978-94-010-9544-0 (eBook)
  DOI 10.1007/978-94-010-9544-0

Contents

□ □ □ □ □ □ □ □ □ □ □ □

Status epilepticus. Febrile convulsions. Childhood seizures.
Rare causes – breath-holding, narcolepsy, metabolic.
Non-epileptic seizures (hysterical).

Nystagmus. Acute vestibular and labyrinthine failure.
Positional vertigo. Ménière's disease. Central vertigo –
multiple sclerosis, vascular disease.
Chronic ataxia – cerebellar signs, cerebellopontine angle
tumours.
Progressive unsteadiness.

Acute – dental, sinusitis, ocular, trauma. Recurrent –
migrainous neuralgia and migrainous variants. Trigeminal neuralgia.
Chronic – compressive causes, post-herpetic neuralgia,
temporo-mandibular joint dysfunction, atypical facial
pain.
Bell's palsy.

Acute visual failure – optic neuritis, ischaemic papillitis.
Transient visual loss. Compression – optic nerve and
chiasm.
Retro-chiasmal pathways. Chronic visual loss – ocular,
compressive, toxic, inherited.
Double vision. Assessment. Ocular motor palsies.
Dysthyroid eye disease. Myasthenia gravis. Conjugate
gaze problems, internuclear ophthalmoplegia, supra-
nuclear palsies. Ocular myopathies.
Proptosis with ophthalmoplegia.

Assessment. Dysphasia. Parietal and frontal lesions.
Brain failure: causes – senile and Alzheimer's dementia,

multi-infarct dementia, normal pressure hydrocephalus.
Search for causes; investigations; management.

writer's cramp, oro-mandibular dystonia. Hemifacial spasm. Restless legs.

Series Editors' Foreword

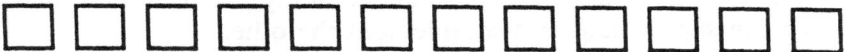

Effective management logically follows accurate diagnosis. Such logic often is difficult to apply in practice. Absolute diagnostic accuracy may not be possible, particularly in the field of primary care, when management has to be on analysis of symptoms and on knowledge of the individual patient and family.

This series follows that on *Problems in Practice* which was concerned more with diagnosis in the widest sense and this series deals more definitively with general care and specific treatment of symptoms and diseases.

Good management must include knowledge of the nature, course and outcome of the conditions, as well as prominent clinical features and assessment and investigations, but the emphasis is on what to do best for the patient.

Family medical practitioners have particular difficulties and advantages in their work. Because they often work in professional isolation in the community and deal with relatively small numbers of near-normal patients their experience with the more serious and more rare conditions is restricted. They find it difficult to remain up-to-date with medical advances and even more difficult to decide on the suitability and application of new and relatively untried methods compared with those that are 'old' and well proven.

Their advantages are that because of long-term continuous care for their patients they have come to know them and their families well and are able to become familiar with the more common and less serious diseases of their communities.

This series aims to correct these disadvantages by providing practical information and advice on the less common, potentially serious conditions, but at the same time to take note of the special features of general medical practice.

To achieve these objectives, the *titles* are intentionally those of accepted body systems and population groups.

The *co-authors* are a specialist and a family practitioner so that each can supplement and complement the other.

The *experience bases* are those of the district general hospital and family practice. It is here that the day-to-day problems arise.

The *advice and presentation* are practical and have come from many years of conjoint experience of family and hospital practice.

The *series* is intended for family practitioners – the young and the less than young. All should benefit and profit from comparing the views of the authors with their own. Many will coincide, some will be accepted as new, useful and worthy of application and others may not be acceptable, but nevertheless will stimulate thought and enquiry.

Since medical care in the community and in hospitals involves teamwork, this series also should be of relevance to nurses and others involved in personal and family care.

JOHN FRY
M. LANCASTER-SMITH

1

Introduction

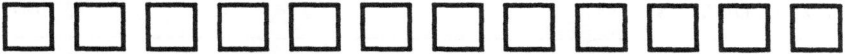

NEUROLOGICAL DISEASE AND THE GENERAL PRACTITIONER

General practitioners are consulted concerning central nervous system (CNS) disease about 75 times a year, slightly more often than for infections of the urinary tract. The annual consulting rates are set out below:

Table 1 Annual patient consulting rates for diseases of central nervous system

Disease	Patients consulting		
	per 1000	per 2500	% of total
Cerebrovascular disorders	6	15	20
Migraine	7	18	24 ⎫
Headaches	4	10	13 ⎬ 37
Vertigo	8	20	26
Epilepsy	3	7	10 ⎫
Parkinsonism	1	3	4 ⎬ 17
Multiple sclerosis	<1	2	3 ⎭
Tumours	0.1	0.25	<1
		(1 in 4 y)	
TOTAL	30	75	100

Only strokes are common. They account for 13% of deaths

1

Table 2 Causes of death in England and Wales 1975 (to nearest 100)

Disease	Number of deaths
Cerebrovascular disease	78 000
Brain tumours and other neoplasms	2 000
Meningitis	300
Multiple sclerosis	800
Parkinsonism	1 600
Epilepsy	600
Motor neurone disease	700
Others	300
All CNS, eye and ear causes	84 300
TOTAL DEATHS	583 000

Tables 1 and 2 are produced by the courtesy of Dr J. Fry and M.T.P. Press[1]

The problems which CNS disease pose the general practitioner are:

(1) The relatively large number of patients presenting with potentially important symptoms, such as headache and vertigo, which demand careful assessment.

(2) The complexity and variety of uncommon but serious disorders of the CNS of which the GP needs to be aware.

(3) The demand upon resources that hypertension and cerebrovascular disease make.

(4) The fear of missing tumours, particularly operable tumours.

(5) The infrequency of contact with neurological problems which render many GPs lacking in confidence.

(6) The variety of therapies available to treat many chronic neurological disorders.

(7) Logistic problems resulting in experienced neurologists and expensive equipment being grouped in centres of excellence.

AN APPROACH TO HISTORY AND EXAMINATION OF THE CNS

A unique position

GPs hold a unique position. They are the first person consulted with a problem, they have knowledge of the patient's premorbid history, social and economic background. They know his personality. They can interview the family and sometimes other witnesses easily. They have access to family histories at first hand. They are well placed to assess drug and alcohol habits. When it comes to rehabilitation, they understand patients' domestic and employment circumstances.

Drugs

Accurate drug records are essential and it is vital that full information is transmitted in referral letters. Dosage, allergies, sensitivity to iodine, knowledge of depressed renal or hepatic function are all important.

Alcohol

The GP is particularly well placed to detect alcoholism. His knowledge of the patient, his frequent contacts with the family, his position of trust and his opportunity for enquiry are second to none. A high index of suspicion is essential coupled with knowledge of at-risk occupations, tell-tale physical and mental symptoms, records of family history and knowledge of personal stresses. Searching via blood tests (MCV, Gamma GT) is legitimate in possible cases, and even challenge with a morning blood sample for alcohol level.

Time dimensions

GPs work in their own time sphere. They can allow problems to unfold, assessing and reassessing at reasonable intervals. It is important that the process is explained to patients and to their relatives and that a phrase such as 'let me know if you are worried' is employed.

A comprehensive examination of the CNS cannot be rushed; it is better to bring the patient back for a long appointment later than to hurry.

General

Examination of the CNS begins with a check through the other systems including the reticulo-endothelial system. In examining the cardiovascular system (CVS) attention should be paid to pulse rhythm, peripheral pulses, presence of bruits at carotids and femorals, lying and standing blood pressure. Neurological symptoms frequently herald the onset of primary tumours in the breast and bronchus and of lymphomas

Higher functions – Check:

Orientation: Time – Space – Person
Speech. Reading. Writing. Spelling. Calculation.
Memory (distant and present): e.g. Name and address recall at one and five minutes.

Motor weakness
Largely discovered by history (see Table 3).

Site	Difficulty
Proximal Arms	Brushing hair, shaving, reaching shelves.
Distal Arms	Keys, buttons, pens.
Proximal Legs	Stairs, low chairs, bath, bed.
Distal Legs	Foot drop – trips up.

Table 3 Motor root innervation of some limb muscles

C 5	Deltoid, Supraspinatus
C 5, 6	Infraspinatus, Biceps, Brachioradialis
C 6, 7	Thenar pad muscles, Flexor pollicis longus
C 6, 7, 8	Triceps, Extensors of wrist and fingers
C 7, 8, T 1	Long finger flexors
C 8, T 1	Small hand muscles, Hypothenar pad muscles
L 1, 2	Ilio-psoas (hip flexors)
L 2, 3, 4	Adductors, Quadriceps
L 4, 5	Tibialis anterior
L 4, 5, S 1	Glutei, Hamstrings
L 5	Extensor hallucis longus
L 5, S 1	Peronei, Soleus, Tibialis posterior, Lateral gastrocnemius
S 1	Medial gastrocnemius, Abductor hallucis
L 5, S 1, 2	Flexor digitorum longus, Flexor hallucis longus

Reflexes

Reflexes are important signs which can be rapidly elicited. The usual root innervations are given in Table 4. Asymmetries are important especially if lateralised. An isolated lost reflex suggests root or peripheral nerve damage; if there is asymptomatic loss of one ankle jerk there may be a past history of sciatica. In older patients (>age 70), lost ankle jerks may suggest a senile neuropathy. Slow relaxation of the ankle jerks may be the first indication of myxoedema.

5

Table 4 Reflexes – Root levels

C 5 } C 6 }	Biceps, Supinator
C 7	Triceps
C 8	Finger
T 8–10	Upper abdominal
T 10–12	Lower abdominal
L 1–2	Cremasteric
L 3–4	Knee
S 1	Ankle

Plantars

The plantar responses are important. A cold foot or very sensitive sole make interpretation difficult. Scratching the lateral border of the sole of a warm foot may help. If the sole is very sensitive, pricking the dorsum of the great toe with a pin causes plantar flexion of the toe in a normal flexor plantar response. If extensor, the toe dorsiflexes trying to impale the pin.

Sensation

Significant sensory loss is often apparent and a patient may accurately show the affected area. This may well correspond to the appropriate territory of a peripheral nerve or root (Figures 1 and 2). Useful dermatome points include C 7 the middle finger, T 4 the nipple, T 10 the umbilicus, L 3 the knee and S 1 the sole. More central disturbances in the sensory pathways may affect different modalities as position sense loss in posterior column disorders, e.g. in tabes, or discriminative functions in parietal lobe upsets. The presence of these pathways also explains how dissociated sensory loss may arise when touch is preserved whilst pain and temperature may be lost, as for example when a syrinx damages the centre of the spinal cord interrupting the crossing spinothalamic fibres but sparing the posterior columns (see Figure 22).

Figure 1 Dermatome distribution in the right arm

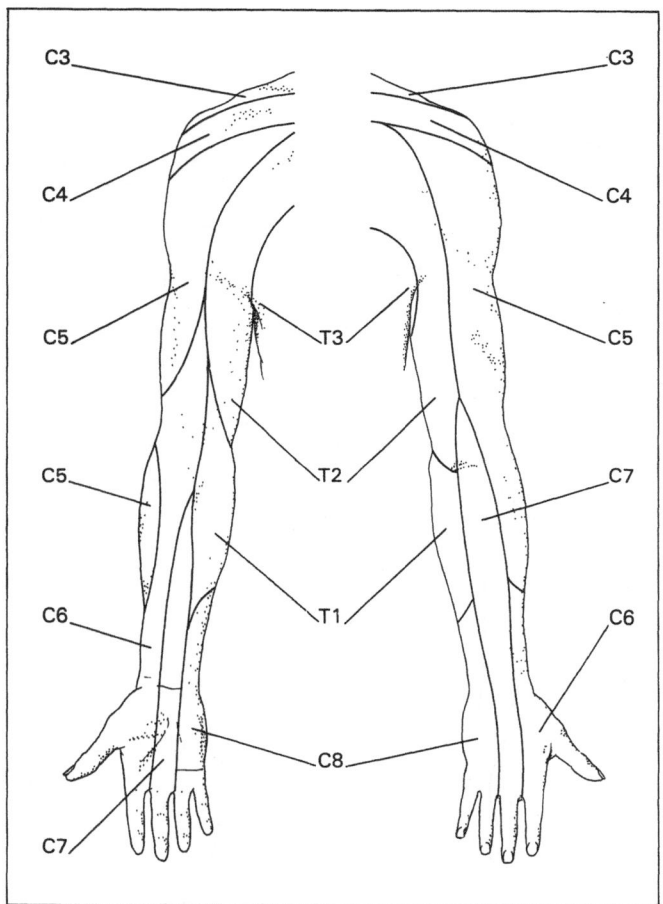

Gait and balance

In patients suspected of any balance or gait disorder, including Parkinson's disease, stance and gait must be examined. Standing on one leg alone or walking around a chair may show a lateralised cerebellar disturbance, while standing tandem – one foot in front

Figure 2 Dermatome distribution in the right leg

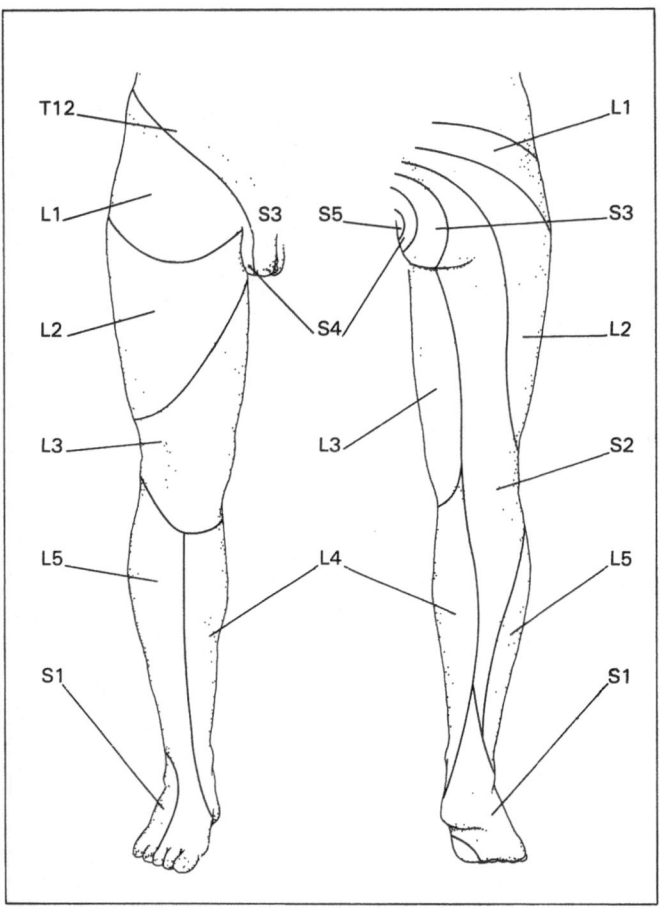

of the other like on a tight-rope, or marking time with the eyes closed, will bring out mild faults of balance (page 64).

The eyes

First measure *visual acuity* using Snellen test type. If patients have a previously unrecognised refractive error or have forgotten their glasses use a pinhole.

For driving, a patient requires an acuity of about 6/12.

Fields Test by confrontation using a small object. A red target (hat pin head) is useful and may show up more subtle areas of field loss by relative impairment of colour intensity in the affected area (see Figures 3 and 4).

Figure 3 Confrontation field testing

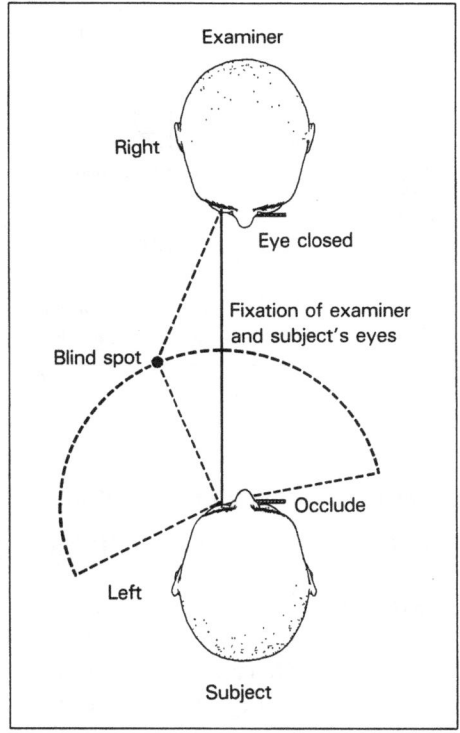

Figure 4 Visual fields

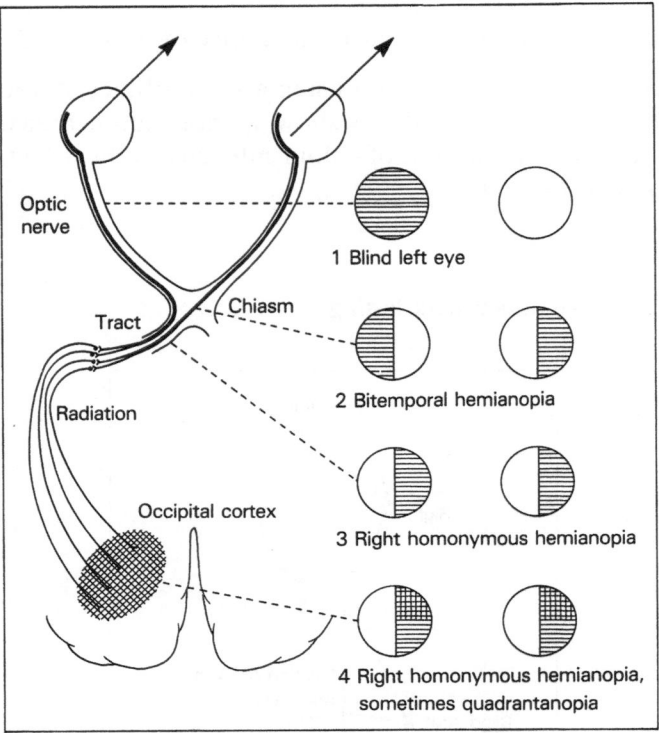

Pupils Test for equality, reaction to light and accommodation.

The principal defects are described in Table 5 and Figure 5.

The afferent pupillary defect In normal patients if the light is swung rapidly from one pupil to the other and back, the pupil will constrict each time, and with repeated stimulation remain constricted. If, however, there is a defect on the afferent pathway of the light reflex (the retina or optic nerve) then there may be paradoxical dilatation of the affected pupil. This is a particularly useful test in patients suspected of an optic neuritis for an afferent defect may be present in the acute phase and also persist after the attack is over.

Ophthalmoscopy A dark room is essential. If there is any difficulty obtaining a well dilated pupil, use a short acting mydriatic (tropicamide 0.5%), unless there is any suspicion of glaucoma.

Examine the retina for haemorrhages, exudates, state of vessels and the presence of nipping at a–v junctions.

Figure 5 Abnormal pupils

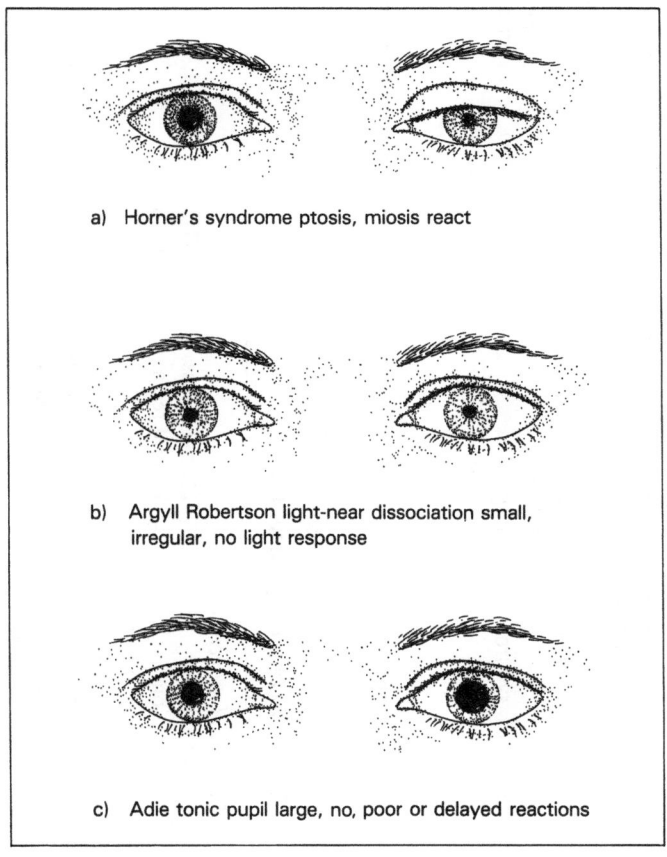

a) Horner's syndrome ptosis, miosis react

b) Argyll Robertson light-near dissociation small, irregular, no light response

c) Adie tonic pupil large, no, poor or delayed reactions

Table 5 Pupils with an abnormal appearance (see also Figure 5)

	Pupil Appearance	Light	Near	Lids	Associated features
(a) Horner's syndrome	small, round unilateral	reacts	reacts	ptosis	sympathetic paralysis central or peripheral
(b) Argyll Robertson	small, irregular bilateral	absent	reacts	slight ptosis	neurosyphilis diabetes occasionally
(c) Adie's syndrome Tonic pupil	large unilateral	absent	slow (tonic)	normal	often absent ankle jerks constricts with weak pilocarpine eye drops 0.125% or mecholyl eye drops 2.5%

Table 6 Action of eye muscles

Horizontal movements
Adduction	Medial rectus	CN3
Abduction	Lateral rectus	CN6

Vertical movements
With the eye abducted

Elevation	Superior rectus	CN3	Extorsion	Inferior oblique	CN3
Depression	Inferior rectus	CN3	Intorsion	Superior oblique	CN4

With the eye adducted

Elevation	Inferior oblique	CN3	Intorsion	Superior rectus	CN3
Depression	Superior oblique	CN4	Extorsion	Inferior rectus	CN3

12

A green light in the ophthalmoscope gives better definition of retinal vessels, haemorrhagic lesions and nerve fibre bundles. Focal atrophy in the nerve fibre layer, as may occur in optic neuritis, may then show as dark slits or grooves.

Examine the disc head. *Papilloedema* is only accompanied by a drop in visual acuity late in the illness although there may be enlargement of the blind spots in the visual fields. A swollen optic disc with marked fall in acuity suggests an optic papillitis, either from inflammation or ischaemia of the nerve head. In early disc swelling there is an absence of venous pulsation in the vessels on the optic disc. The presence of pulsation is against a diagnosis of papilloedema.

Eye movements The range of eye movements from side to side and up and down are also important. These should be tested to command and then with the patient following an object. Disordered eye movements in which the two eyes are not yoked in parallel, dysconjugate, may arise from a central (brain stem) or peripheral fault (cranial nerve or ocular muscle). An amblyopic eye or a longstanding fault often produces no symptoms but any recent ocular imbalance causes diplopia.

In assessing diplopia it is necessary to check whether the separation of images is horizontal or vertical, and in which direction of gaze the separation of the two images is maximal.

The action of the eye muscles is set out in Table 6.

A complete oculomotor palsy produces an abducted eye with no significant other movement, complete ptosis with the lid covering the whole eye, and an enlarged pupil (Figure 11).

Often limitation of the range of eye movement indicates which muscles are paretic. However, the other useful aid in assessing the site of a peripheral muscle weakness causing diplopia is the *cover test*. Here the patient is asked to look in the direction of gaze that causes maximal separation of the two images. Each eye is covered in turn and the more peripheral image noted. The eye from which the most peripheral image arises has the weak muscle. Further details are given in Chapter 6.

Nystagmus Nystagmus describes small involuntary jerky movements of the eyes. There is usually a fast and slow phase and the direction of jerk nystagmus is given by the direction of the fast phase. Nystagmus can be elicited in normal patients looking at a moving target. Fine horizontal nystagmus is most often due to a peripheral labyrinthine disturbance (this is often suppressed by fixation) or to drugs. Vertical or rotary nystagmus or very coarse nystagmus usually suggests a central origin in the brain stem or its connections. Occasionally nystagmus may make a patient aware of objects moving, oscillopsia. Further details are given in Chapter 4.

INVESTIGATIONS

Many neurological investigations are invasive procedures carrying a small but definite risk and GPs may be asked details about these by their patients. Simple routine blood tests and X-rays require little explanation. An EEG is non-invasive, usually done as an out-patient procedure, but does require co-operation with a relatively still patient. Visual and auditory evoked potentials (VEPs and AEPs) involve surface scalp recordings from pad electrodes after either a visual (alternating checker-board flashing pattern) or auditory (click) stimulus. Electromyography (EMG) involves the sampling of a number of muscles with a fine needle. The muscle activity is measured at rest and during contraction. This is combined with the measurement of nerve conduction velocity and action potential amplitude which requires electrical stimulation of limb nerves. Some patients find this uncomfortable.

Radiological investigations include CT brain scanning, similar to an X-ray, which is commonly performed on out-patients. However, patients must be co-operative enough to lie still during the procedure. The pictures may be repeated after an intravenous (IV) injection of iodine-containing contrast media. This may produce nausea and vomiting in a few patients, and rarely, a more severe allergic reaction to the iodine.

Lumbar puncture is used to obtain cerebrospinal fluid (CSF) for examination: this is essential in patients suspected of meningitis or sub-arachnoid haemorrhage. It is often helpful in the diagnosis of other conditions as multiple sclerosis (MS) or acute polyneuritis. Lumbar puncture is also used as the means for the introduction of radio-opaque media, isotopes or air for neuroradiological diagnosis (myelography, cisternography, pneumo-encephalography). About 20–25% of patients develop a low pressure headache post-puncture eased by lying and aggravated by standing. This occasionally lasts days. Rarely, cranial nerve palsies may follow a lumbar puncture. It is dangerous to perform a lumbar puncture (LP) in the presence of an intracranial mass as this may provoke a pressure cone with brain shifts causing compression either at the tentorial hiatus or at the foramen magnum. These are life-threatening. LP is also contraindicated in the presence of local skin sepsis.

If cord compression is suspected in the spinal canal myelography will be performed. This involves the injection of radio-opaque iodine containing contrast into the lumbar theca below the termination of the spinal cord. The dye now most commonly used is water-soluble and disappears quickly. After the procedure the patient sits up for some hours and about 25% may develop unpleasant vomiting, head and backache usually settling after the next 48 hours. Very rarely more alarming neurological sequelae may appear. Myodil (Pantopaque), an oily dye, was the contrast medium used formerly. This had a small risk of producing an arachnoiditis so that many doctors advise its removal after the procedure. This involves another LP and the aspiration of as much contrast as is possible, and is often uncomfortable.

Angiography requires arterial puncture with the injection of iodine-containing contrast. This may be done by direct needle puncture in the carotid artery in the neck or more commonly via a catheter introduced into a distant artery, often the femoral. Many such procedures are done under general anaesthetic (GA). Again such patients may prove allergic to the contrast and the arterial puncture carries a risk, particularly in arteriopaths, so there is a morbidity, most commonly the production of a stroke, and even a very small mortality (less than 1 in 200). Spinal angiography is used to show the circulation of the spinal cord. Here selective catheterisation is performed on the feeding arterial branches. Rarely this may provoke transient spasms or even cord damage.

Air-encephalography (AEG, pneumo-encephalography) has largely been replaced by CT scanning. An LP is performed and air injected into the sub-arachnoid space. The air introduced passes up into the ventricles in the brain and by altering the position of the patient can be moved about to outline these cavities. Such procedures usually provoke intense headache and there is a morbidity particularly in the presence of a mass lesion. If a supratentorial mass is suspected then air or sometimes contrast media may be introduced into the ventricles directly using a cannula inserted through a burr hole, ventriculography.

All these invasive investigations are done as in-patient procedures.

HOSPITAL ADMISSION

Urgent for all patients:

- – in coma
- – suspected of meningitis

    cerebral abscess

    encephalitis

    sub-arachnoid haemorrhage
- – with status epilepticus or serial major seizures
- – with bulbar or respiratory muscle weakness as in polio, myasthenia gravis, polyneuritis, tetanus
- – with polyneuritis of acute onset and rapid progression
- – suspected of spinal cord compression or root involvement with rapid (days) progressive limb weakness, sensory loss and/or sphincter upset

16

- suspected of raised intracranial pressure from a mass lesion with deteriorating conscious level and/or progressive focal signs
- with acutely progressive visual loss (over days)
- with head injuries with either loss of consciousness (5 minutes or more), significant amnesia or both
- with a deteriorating or fluctuating conscious level of unknown cause
- with acute severe headache and neurological or ocular signs.

Admission is commonly required in most patients:

- with acute severe headache (unless recurrent); some of these will prove to be a first migraine attack
- with suspected acute strokes
- with toxic confusional states
- with intractable root or spinal pain
- with progressive limb weakness or other focal signs
- with significant neurological disability which cannot be managed at home, e.g. an acute relapse in MS, end-stage Parkinson's disease
- undergoing more detailed neurological investigation, e.g. myelography, angiography.

To some extent the age and previous physical state of the patient may influence the decision. Children and young, previously healthy, adults will merit more aggressive management. Urgent out–patient referrals or domiciliary consultations may be possible in the management of some patients in the second group.

2

Headache

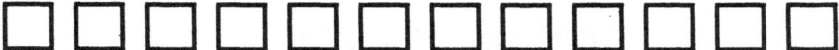

Headache is the most common neurological symptom. It is the most frequent cause of complaints of pain and over one third of GP consultations for neurological disorders are for headache. These headaches most commonly are the result of migraine and muscle contraction, or tension, but serious causes as meningitis, intracranial bleeding or masses need consideration. In one series of consultations for headache, however, only one patient in 65 showed a serious cause[2].

ANATOMY

In the head and face only certain structures are pain sensitive. These include the skin and muscles of the scalp, the periosteum of the skull, parts of the dura, the surfaces lining the tentorium, the walls of the large arteries and veins and some local structures – eyes, teeth, sinuses, jaw joints.

The top of the head, face and supratentorial intracranial compartment are innervated by the trigeminal nerves. The infratentorial compartment (posterior fossa), back of the head and neck are innervated by the second and third cervical roots, and by branches of the vagus and glossopharyngeal nerves. These last two may cause pain referred to the ear and throat.

PAIN PRODUCTION

The pain of headache is usually produced by[3]:
(1)   Meningeal irritation by infection or blood.
(2)   Raised intracranial pressure (ICP).
(3)   Traction, distension or compression of intra- and extracranial blood vessels.
(4)   Irritation, stretching or compression of sensory nerves.
(5)   Muscle spasm (commonly of the scalp and neck).

PROBLEMS THE GP MUST CONSIDER

(1)   Why does the patient present with headache now?
(2)   Is it serious?
(3)   How does the patient expect the doctor to deal with it?
(4)   When is it necessary to refer the patient to hospital?
(5)   What is the likely natural history?
(6)   What is the scope for 'cure'?

HISTORY

It is useful to have a scheme to follow in taking the history; that suggested by Lance[4] is effective. In most instances patients show no abnormal signs so the history is all important. A number of points are emphasised.

(1)   The *length* of history – headaches heralding more serious disease usually have a short duration whereas headaches of more than one year's duration seldom have any serious cause, unless there has been a change in pattern.

(2)   The *frequency* of attacks and their *duration*. There is an obvious difference between recurrent attacks, which are often migrainous, and chronic continuous headache as may occur with muscle contraction.

20

(3) The *site* and *quality* of the pain – often a brief sketch of the site and any radiation is a help. Throbbing or pulsatile pain suggests a vascular or inflammatory cause.

(4) The *mode of onset* and any *associated features,* e.g. vomiting or visual upset.

(5) *Precipitating* or *aggravating causes* and any measures that afford *relief*. When there is raised ICP, any manoeuvre which increases the pressure further will increase the pain. This includes coughing, sneezing, bending, and exertion. Headache actually awakening patients from sleep should be taken seriously. It should also be remembered that sometimes pain is referred from the eyes, teeth or infected sinuses.

RECURRENT HEADACHE

Migraine

Definition This causes attacks of lateralised headache, hemicrania, associated with nausea and vomiting (c.90%) and prostration. The site of the pain, its intensity, frequency and duration may vary considerably. In some, the pain is generalised, in others centred in one orbit or even spreads into the face and neck.

Frequency Migraine is very common, probably affecting some 10% of men, some 20% of women and some 10% of children. There is usually a family history, particularly in childhood migraine. There also appears to be an association with travel sickness.

Course Many patients have two to four attacks yearly, others have clusters of frequent attacks interspersed with long periods of freedom, and a few show increasing repeated episodes, status migrainosus. A number of patients find their attacks cease as they get older.

What is it? In many patients there is a warning said to reflect vasoconstriction of the affected vessel and this produces transient ischaemic symptoms. These are often visual with flashing lights, zig-zags, odd patterns, scotomata, field loss or disturbed focus.

Giddiness may occur in some 25%. More alarming symptoms include a hemiparesis (in 5%), hemisensory upsets (often brachiofacial in distribution), speech disturbances, double vision or even loss of consciousness. Such warning symptoms usually last 15 – 45 minutes and are followed by the build-up of an intense throbbing headache. This is thought due to vasodilatation and the pain usually lasts hours, occasionally one or two days. The headache is aggravated by light in 80% and many patients dislike noise. Vomiting or sleep may relieve the headache. In about 20% there may be a loose bowel action.

Children Children with migraine may present with recurrent sick headaches but there is also a significant group who present with central abdominal pain (at the umbilicus), nausea and vomiting and sometimes headache. It is possible some children with so-called 'grumbling appendices' may have abdominal migraine. Such children usually appear pale, floppy and lethargic in an attack. They may describe visual symptoms, distorted body image, speech upset, limb pains or tingling and photophobia. There is commonly a strongly positive family history.

Between attacks patients show no abnormal signs but in the attack there may be photophobia, scalp tenderness and even dilated scalp vessels.

Triggers Many triggers are recognised. These include:
(1) Certain food substances – chocolate, cheese, citrus fruit, onions, highly spiced foods, Chinese food (monosodium glutamate) and cured meat (nitrites).
(2) Hypoglycaemia – fasting or missed meals.
(3) Hormones – menstruation, the contraceptive pill, the menopause.
(4) Trauma – head injuries (footballers' migraine).
(5) Exertion.
(6) Fever – intercurrent infections.
(7) Alcohol – particularly red wine and spirits.
(8) Travel.

(9) Sleep – excess or missed.

(10) Stress and stress-release – Saturday morning headache.

Contraceptive pill Women taking the oral contraceptive pill who are migrainous subjects have an increased incidence of thrombotic strokes. If a patient taking the 'pill' develops migrainous attacks or finds their established migrainous attacks change their pattern, then they should stop the 'pill'.

Complex Rarely, vascular damage in the brain or retina may occur in a severe migraine attack. In *ophthalmoplegic migraine* there is an oculomotor palsy. In *hemiplegic migraine* a hemiparesis may appear. With time most of these deficits may disappear. Other migrainous variants are discussed in Chapter 5.

Symptomatic Occasionally attacks may be symptomatic, often of a vascular lesion, such as an angioma or meningioma. Here the attacks are always in the territory of the affected vessel and there are often focal neurological signs. Patients with acute intense prostrating headache with abnormal signs, particularly if in the first attack, will usually need admission to hospital.

Management

This depends on the frequency and severity of attacks. Most migraine sufferers manage their own attacks but explanation and reassurance prove helpful. All recognised triggers should be avoided. There is no 'cure' for migraine.

In the first severe attack the diagnosis may be uncertain. In the young, alarming symptoms may develop rapidly and in older patients with complex attacks referral is often necessary to exclude other causes.

Treatment In adults a simple analgesic – soluble aspirin 600–900 mg or soluble paracetamol 1 g, taken as early as possible – may be effective. In migraine, absorption of drugs is delayed and if a patient is nauseated or has vomited, oral preparations may be ineffective. Tablets of metoclopramide (Maxolon) 10 mg, will help relieve nausea and aid absorption of analgesics. With severe vomiting a suppository of prochlorperazine (Stemetil) 25 mg may be useful. There are also a number of proprietary preparations where an analgesic and anti-emetic are combined.

Ergot A proportion of patients in the acute attack may be helped by ergotamine, a potent vasoconstrictor, taking 1 – 2 mg early in the attack. Other oral preparations include Lingraine (2 mg of ergotamine), Cafergot (1 mg of ergotamine with 100 mg of caffeine) and Migril (2 mg ergotamine, 100 mg of caffeine and 50 mg cyclizine). There is also an ergotamine inhaler (about 0.36 mg per puff) and Cafergot suppositories (2 mg ergotamine and 100 mg caffeine). These last may be useful if there is severe nausea or early vomiting. A number of patients, however, find ergot derivatives upset them, causing nausea and vomiting. Furthermore it is possible to become habituated to ergot with the development of dependent headache, so a cycle of recurring headaches only relieved by the next dose of ergot may arise. In excessive dosage, ergot poisoning (ergotism), may occur with the development of limb ischaemia and even gangrene. Ergotamine may aggravate angina and should be avoided in pregnancy.

Prevention (interval treatment)

In two thirds of migrainous patients the frequency and severity of attacks may be reduced by the regular intake of a number of preparations. These will be necessary if the frequency of attacks is more than three per month. If successful the treatment should be continued for three months and then discontinued to assess the effect. Interval preparations include:

(1) *Pizotifen* (Sanomigran) 0.5 mg b.d. increasing to 1.5 mg b.d. This is a serotonin antagonist and usually well tolerated. It may cause weight gain and drowsiness.

(2) *Propranolol* (Inderal) 20 mg b.d. increasing to 80 mg t.i.d. if necessary. This is a beta-blocker probably maintaining vasoconstriction. It should not be given to patients with any

history of asthma, obstructive airways disease or heart failure. It has a slow onset of action and the dose needs to be built up slowly. It may provoke nausea, vivid dreams, faint feelings and cold extremities.

(3) *Methysergide* (Deseril) 1 mg b.d. increasing to 2 mg t.i.d. This also blocks the action of serotonin. Rarely it has caused retroperitoneal fibrosis and so it should not be given in continuous courses for longer than 16 weeks without a pause of one to two months. It may also cause insomnia and depression and is best avoided in patients with a history of peptic ulceration or ischaemic heart disease.

(4) *Clonidine* (Dixarit) 50 micrograms b.d. increasing to 75 micrograms b.d. This inhibits noradrenaline release and in the author's hands has not proved very effective. It may cause a dry mouth, drowsiness and depression.

(5) *Prochlorperazine* (Stemetil) 5 mg t.i.d. This is a phenothiazine and may be useful if giddiness is prominent in the attack. It may cause drowsiness and even an acute dystonic reaction, particularly in young women or girls.

(6) *Tricyclic anti-depressants* These may be helpful particularly if depression, anxiety or insomnia are part of the background. Often a single dose given at bed-time is helpful, e.g. amitriptyline 50–150 mg, dothiepin (Prothiaden) 25–75 mg, or trimipramine (Surmontil) 25–75 mg. These may cause a dry mouth, drowsiness, rashes or aggravate constipation, urinary retention or glaucoma.

(7) *Benzodiazepines* may be helpful in short courses if anxiety is troublesome.

Children In acute attacks a simple analgesic given as early as possible is often the best. If attacks are very frequent and severe, then pizotifen 0.5 mg increasing to 1 mg nocte is effective. Other substances worth a trial include promethazine hydrochloride (Phenergan) 10–25 mg nocte (depending on age) and even propranolol.

SERIOUS CAUSES OF HEADACHE

Headache provoked by *meningeal irritation* either from infection or bleeding has a short history with intense pain, commonly frontal or generalised, often throbbing in quality. With infection the headache builds up accompanied by drowsiness. In sub-arachnoid haemorrhage (SAH) the sudden onset is characteristic so that sometimes patients imagine they have been struck a blow. In a number they may actually fall or lose consciousness. Headache from haemorrhage may follow exertion or stress.

Such headaches are associated with meningism – a stiff neck and restricted straight leg raising (Kernig's sign). Rarely in the very young, the very old or in immune-compromised patients, meningism may be absent. Some patients complain of backache.

Such patients appear ill, febrile and are photophobic. Often they are drowsy, confused, irritable and resent examination. They may show nausea, vomiting and loss of appetite. Some patients have focal neurological signs – limb or facial weakness, oculomotor palsies and even papilloedema. Some may present with epileptic seizures. Transient glycosuria may occur after a haemorrhage.

Relief from the headache is often obtained by lying in a darkened room and simple analgesics, as aspirin or paracetamol, will reduce the pain and any fever.

Such patients require *admission* to hospital urgently so the CSF can be examined. Delay in making the diagnosis and starting treatment in meningitis increases the mortality and morbidity.

RAISED INTRACRANIAL PRESSURE (ICP) BRAIN TUMOURS

The headache of raised pressure is again commonly of short duration, building up over a few days or weeks. It is often episodic and may be localised or generalised. If sited at the back of the head it may reflect a posterior fossa mass and this sometimes may displace the cerebellar tonsils into the foramen magnum, tonsillar herniation, producing a stiff neck. With raised ICP the pain is worse on waking and may be precipitated or aggravated by exercise or any measures causing a further pressure rise, e.g. opening the bowels, straining, sexual intercourse. Often there is associated nausea and vomiting. Lesions near the floor of the fourth ventricle are particularly likely to cause vomiting and sometimes hiccup. If the pressure is very high with severe swelling of the optic discs, then a patient may develop transient obscurations of vision often triggered by bending or exertion. This is an ominous sign, for if not heeded, visual impairment or even blindness can follow.

Signs In many patients with raised ICP from a mass there will be depression of the conscious level with drowsiness, and often focal neurological signs but only a proportion will show papilloedema. In children with headache from brain tumour nearly 90% show abnormal neurological or ocular signs. Relatives may comment on changes in personality or behaviour and there may be unsteadiness. In addition to focal signs associated directly with the site of a mass there may be *false localising signs* from the elevated pressure – for example an abducens palsy may appear causing diplopia.

Some supratentorial masses may cause herniation of mid-brain structures through the tentorial hiatus with impairment of upgaze and the development of an oculomotor palsy often shown first by an enlarging pupil with impaired light reaction. If this pressure cone is allowed to continue then the patient will become unconscious with fixed dilated pupils and lost brain stem reflexes. This state may produce irreversible damage.

Headache with loss of consciousness Occasionally patients with an intermittent obstructive hydrocephalus may present with attacks of crescendo headache. These arise acutely and at the height of the headache the patient may fall to the ground unconscious, usually for a short period. Some show a slower recovery. Obstructive hydrocephalus is often accompanied by dementia and papilloedema.

It is always worth checking the scalp of patients suspected of raised ICP for any signs of local infection, recent trauma or swellings.

Cough headache Cough headache may reflect the presence of a posterior fossa mass, raised ICP, a hydrocephalus or even arise as a benign entity. It is always worth taking seriously.

Patients suspected of raised ICP require referral to hospital for further investigation, many as a matter of urgency. This is imperative if there is a depressed conscious level, stiff neck, fever or progressive focal signs.

GIANT CELL ARTERITIS (GCA), TEMPORAL OR CRANIAL ARTERITIS

This produces an acute patchy inflammation of arteries, commonly of the scalp – external carotid branches, but also of intracranial branches and of retinal vessels. The inflammation may set up a thrombotic endarteritis with occlusion of the affected artery and if this is a vessel supplying the retina or optic nerve may lead to *blindness*. If arteries supplying cranial nerves or the brain are affected, this may produce an ophthalmoplegia or stroke.

GCA affects elderly patients, 60 years and over, and is associated with malaise, joint pains, night sweats, weight loss and impaired appetite. Younger patients may be affected by a vasculitis but this is usually part of a polyarteritis nodosa with more widespread manifestations. There is a high incidence of GCA in patients with polymyalgia rheumatica.

Characteristically an elderly patient develops acute distressing headache, often throbbing and persistent in nature. The pain may cause night awakening and there is usually local tenderness over affected scalp vessels, most often the temporal arteries. This may cause pain on chewing and patients dislike brushing their hair. The affected artery may feel swollen and thickened.

In such patients an ESR should be set up immediately. If this is elevated, >60 mm/hour, then without delay steroid treatment should be started, prednisolone 60–80 mg/day. This is to prevent any thrombotic episode with irreversible visual loss. If the diagnosis is correct, within 24–48 hours the patient will have responded to treatment. Many patients are referred to hospital to confirm the diagnosis. Here an arterial biopsy may be performed and it is important to choose a clinically affected artery.

Patients with GCA require continuing treatment with steroids for some time. Progress is usually monitored clinically and with the ESR level. An initial dose of prednisolone 60–80 mg/day may be reduced every seven to ten days by 20 mg/day providing there is no further ESR rise. Most patients are then maintained on a low dose of steroids (5–10 mg/day of prednisolone) for at least twelve months, but if there is any suspicion of a return of activity or a rising ESR, then the dose may need further increase.

CHRONIC HEADACHE

It is always reassuring to know that in a series of 1152 patients with chronic headache (pain present for over one year), only one was found to have a cerebral tumour; 612 patients had migraine and 466 tension headache[5].

Chronic persistent headache recurring daily over many months or years usually reflects *muscle contraction, tension,* with sometimes added depression. The pain is usually present throughout the waking hours fluctuating in severity. In many it is described as a tight band, a weight, heaviness or pressure around, over or in the head. In 90% it is bilateral. It is often described in superlatives yet sufferers are able to work or run a home normally.

The pain does not interfere with sleep but some patients notice its presence on waking. If it actually awakens the patient from sleep, then other causes should be considered. In about a quarter of patients the pain at times appears throbbing, suggesting a mixture of tension and migraine.

Nearly 75% of patients are women. The pain may have been present for many years. In some there are also complaints of giddiness, faint feelings and impaired concentration.

Lateralised muscle contraction pain centred in one temple and aggravated by chewing, raises the possibility of temporomandibular joint (TMJ) dysfunction.

Change of pattern Beware of patients with chronic headache in whom the pattern of the pain changes. This may introduce all the causes of more acute headache some of which are serious.

Patients with tension headache show no abnormal signs. In a few, obvious muscle spasm and tightness can be found. Some patients are *depressed*. A number of middle aged and older patients may show restriction in their range of neck movements which may be associated with a degree of cervical spondylosis (*q.v.*).

Investigations In older patients a full blood count, ESR (arteritis) and X-rays of the skull (pineal shift, abnormal calcification, eroded sella), chest (lung cancer) and sometimes cervical spine (spondylosis) may be helpful.

Management Treatment of chronic headache is difficult. Reassurance and explanation are very important. Time may be well spent discussing any possible stress, giving relief to pent-up emotions, and dealing with any fears expressed. In many patients, particularly if there is any element of depression, a single dose tricyclic anti-depressant given at bed-time helps. If sleep is poor trimipramine (Surmontil) 25–75 mg nocte is useful, or if anxiety is prominent dothiepin (Prothiaden) 25–75 mg nocte can be tried. It is best to be familiar with one or two tricyclic compounds, knowing their indications, dose range and side effects. In a few patients there may be an obvious gain from their persistent headache. Fluctuations of severe pain may be helped by simple analgesics but addicting compounds as dihydrocodeine (DF118) should be avoided.

A few patients benefit from hypnosis, self-relaxation, neck exercises or acupuncture, which may also help some migraine sufferers.

CERVICAL SPONDYLOSIS

Degenerative changes occur in the vertebral joints in the cervical spine in most patients as they age. Such changes are apparent on the X-rays of most older patients. However, in only a proportion do these seem associated with pain usually radiating from the neck into the occipital region, in the distribution of the second and third cervical roots. Sometimes this pain appears to spread over the head. It commonly appears associated with muscle spasm. Rarely such patients may also have symptoms and signs to suggest cervical root involvement with complaints of pain or sensory upset in the arms (page 130).

The acute pain and spasm may be helped by analgesics, muscle relaxants, support in a cervical collar, and heat and physiotherapy.

POST-TRAUMATIC HEADACHE

Headache following *head injury* is common. It is easy to think that intracranial bruising with meningeal irritation may provoke this. Furthermore, trauma may sometimes aggravate or precipitate migraine.

However, in some patients with seemingly minor head injuries there may be complaints of persistent, severe headache often far in excess of what is expected. This is particularly likely if there is any compensation issue.

Post-concussive Concussive injuries will certainly provoke dizziness, light headedness, blurred vision, impaired concentration, irritability and depressed libido (page 194). In such patients sophisticated balance tests (caloric tests and electronystagmography) will demonstrate disturbances in the balance pathways. Psychometric tests on patients with a post-traumatic amnesia of more than 24 hours usually show changes for the worse – all supporting an organic basis in many patients.

The exact mechanism of the headache is difficult although in many features the pattern resembles muscle contraction pain. The pain is very variable – aching, pressing, throbbing, stabbing, band-like. It is often aggravated by exertion or mental effort and relieved by rest. In some, natural fear of brain damage may in part be responsible, in others the pain pattern suggests this may be arising from blood vessels.

Management Examination should reveal no abnormal neurological signs. Often referral is made to a specialist particularly where there is a medico-legal claim. In adults a skull X-ray may be useful.

31

50% of normal patients will show a central calcified pineal on the films. Displacement of this in patients with post-traumatic headache raises the question of a subdural haematoma. However, the haematoma may be bilateral or the pineal may not be calcified.

In most patients with post-traumatic headache the pain settles in time. Initial rest, reassurance and simple analgesics are helpful. Persistent pain usually requires specialist referral.

SUBDURAL HAEMATOMA

This is due to an intracranial clot in the subdural space. Commonly it arises from traumatic tearing of the surface veins and may occur acutely or more slowly. Subsequently the 'clot' may expand progressively compressing the brain. It is more frequent in the *elderly*; two thirds arise in patients over 50. In such patients the veins are more fragile and the brain more atrophic. Subdural haematoma (SDH) is more common in patients receiving anti-coagulants, in chronic alcoholics, and in those with intracranial surgical shunts. Chronic SDH may also occur in infancy.

Symptoms There is usually a complaint of dull generalised headache present for several weeks, associated with impaired alertness, apathy and often faulty memory. The last may cause some patients to forget the injury that produced the clot. Sometimes the headache may have features of elevated ICP, and even appear worse on lying down. Many patients show *fluctuating symptoms* and signs. Some present with a confusional state or even dementia.

In about one third of patients there may be papilloedema. Most patients appear drowsy, although this may be intermittent. They are often vague and muddled. Commonly there is impairment of upgaze, occasionally pupillary inequality, focal limb weakness and even an extensor plantar response. In about one third of patients the SDH may be bilateral. In some patients with a unilateral clot and a calcified pineal gland, displacement of the latter on skull X-ray may give the diagnosis.

32

Patients suspected of SDH should be referred to hospital. CT brain scanning is the investigation of choice, but a few clots are iso-dense and if bilateral may prove difficult to recognise.

OTHER HEADACHES

Some headaches, particularly chronic, defy recognition or placing into any single clear category. They may be very varied but often include brief episodes of sharp or stabbing scalp pains. Some of these may be migrainous variants (page 80) and may even respond to specific treatment such as indomethacin. Such patients are usually referred to hospital where also they prove difficult to label. However, the absence of abnormal signs may at least reassure the doctor.

REFERRED PAINS

Headache may also arise from:

(1) *Sinus infection* Here the pain is often in the frontal region, around the eyes, or in the cheek depending on which sinus is involved, or if this is a pansinusitis. There is a blocked or stuffy nose, purulent catarrh and often local tenderness. The pain may throb and be aggravated by bending (page 77).

(2) *Ocular pain* This may occur with local inflammation of the conjunctiva, cornea or iris. The eye is usually reddened, may feel gritty and there may be visual blurring. The pain is usually well localised to the affected eye (page 77). *Acute glaucoma* from a rise in intraocular pressure produces a steady aching pain in the eye, sometimes spreading into the orbit and frontal region. The conjunctiva is injected and the acuity depressed. The eyeball may be tender.

Prolonged close work in patients with hypermetropia and astigmatism without correction may produce muscle contraction pain, often in the frontal region.

33

(3) *Dental pain* With infection or an abscess, pain may spread from the face into the frontal region. Usually local tenderness of the affected tooth and other features of local inflammation point to these causes (page 76).

SYSTEMIC ILLNESSES

Headache may occur in many systemic illnesses:

(1) with fever, e.g. 'flu', mumps

(2) with hypercapnia, e.g. in chronic obstructive airways disease

(3) from drugs, e.g. glyceryl trinitrate or other vasodilators

(4) from carbon monoxide poisoning.

A number of patients with *hypertension* may develop headache although most patients in the early stages are symptomless. In some, the pain has the features of a vascular mechanism and responds to the control of the blood pressure. In others, muscle contraction pain, perhaps linked with anxiety, is likely to be the mechanism. Patients with an acute rise in blood pressure as may occur while taking monoamine oxidase inhibitors together with cheese or alcohol, or the rare patient with a pheochromocytoma, may develop sudden intense prostrating headache often aggravated by lying flat. In a few such patients a sub-arachnoid haemorrhage may occur.

MANAGEMENT OF PATIENTS WITH ESTABLISHED CEREBRAL TUMOURS

GPs may help in the management of patients with confirmed cerebral tumours. These may be gliomas, proven by biopsy or after partial excision, or more commonly multiple metastases (particularly from the lung, breast, kidney, alimentary tract, thyroid and melanoma). Some patients may have received radiotherapy and many are already taking steroids (often dexamethasone). Most benign tumours will have been excised unless the patient is too old or too unfit.

Dexamethasone (and other steroids) are effective in temporarily reducing oedema around a cerebral tumour and particularly around metastases. A high dose is used initially (e.g. dexamethasone 12–16 mg/day) and this reduced to a low level (often 2–4 mg/daily) to try and control symptoms of raised intracranial pressure – headache, drowsiness, and also focal symptoms as weakness. Some patients may be maintained on such palliative measures with, if necessary, analgesics and anti-emetics for weeks or even months. High dose steroids, however, for any duration produce side effects. Anti-convulsants may also be necessary.

Such patients terminally become slower and more drowsy. If pain is severe and distressing they may need regular doses of strong analgesics (DDAs). Relatives may wish to nurse such patients at home but often they will need a final hospital admission.

3

Loss of Consciousness

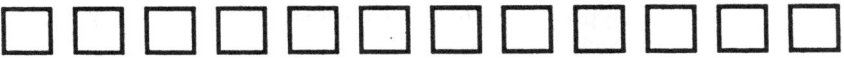

LOSS OF CONSCIOUSNESS (LOC)

In the diagnosis of episodes of LOC the account of an eye-witness is the most important single aid. Where this is not available, then the account from the patient may help. The two common causes of LOC are *faints* (syncope, vasovagal attacks) and *epileptic seizures* (fits). Others are included in Table 7. *Syncope* LOC from a vascular mechanism produces a fall in cerebral perfusion. This has a slow onset with often faint feelings, nausea, headache, dimming of vision and hearing. The attacks start with the patient in an upright position and the aftermath is not prolonged.

The circumstances of a faint may be very relevant: standing in a hot, crowded room, the sight of blood, pain, a distressing experience, getting up after a spell in bed, blood loss, dehydration. Commonly there is warning and recovery is usually rapid.

The pulse is weak and slow and the patient appears pale, sometimes this being accompanied by a cold sweat. It is uncommon for injury to occur.

A problem arises in that sometimes a more prolonged episode of *cerebral anoxia* may provoke *seizure features*. If the cerebral circulation is impaired for twenty seconds or more, then there may be rigidity, twitching, eye rolling and incontinence. This most often

Table 7 Causes of transient loss of consciousness or loss of awareness

(1) *Vascular*
- (i) Faints, syncope, vasodepressor episodes
  - a) simple
  - b) cough
  - c) micturition
- (ii) Carotid sinus sensitivity
- (iii) Postural hypotension   drugs
       autonomic neuropathy –
       diabetes
- (iv) Abnormalities of heart rate or rhythm
  - a) heart block   Stokes–Adams
  - b) supraventricular tachycardia
  - c) 'sick' sinus syndrome
- (v) Abnormalities of cardiac filling or output
  - a) aortic stenosis
  - b) Valsalva's manoeuvre
  - c) atrial myxoma
  - d) myocardial infarct
- (vi) Vertebro-basilar insufficiency
  - a) basilar migraine
  - b) vertebro-basilar ischaemia
- (vii) Transient global amnesia

(2) *Metabolic*
- (i) Hypoglycaemia
- (ii) Hypocalcaemia
- (iii) Hyperventilation

(3) *Trauma*

(4) *Epilepsy*
- (i) Generalised
  - a) grand mal, tonic–clonic
  - b) petit mal, absences
  - c) myoclonic
  - d) others – akinetic, salaam attacks
- (ii) Partial (focal) *
  - a) simple   motor, Jacksonian
         sensory
  - b) complex   temporal lobe
  - *some partial seizures become generalised

(5) *Hysteria*
Non-epileptic seizures

follows a faint where the patient remains upright – wedged in a chair, or held erect by well-wishers.

VARIANTS

Coughing in prolonged paroxysms may interfere with venous return to the heart and stimulate baroceptors causing a fall in cardiac output with syncope. It most often affects men with chronic obstructive airways disease who are smokers.

Micturition syncope occurs in middle aged or older men at night who are emptying or have just emptied their bladders. The explanation is uncertain but thought to be due to vasodilatation of blood vessels in the legs. The advice to empty the bladder at night sitting down will prevent attacks.

Carotid sinus syncope is due to sensitivity of the carotid sinus in the neck to pressure, as from a tight collar. This causes faint feelings or LOC from temporary asystole. Patients should always be tested lying down and care should be given in the elderly not to provoke any prolonged episode.

Cardiac causes of LOC are well recognised. An acute myocardial infarct may present in this way when the heart as a pump fails. There may also be a failure of cardiac output from inflow obstruction, as with a Valsalva manoeuvre or atrial myxoma, or outflow obstruction, as with a tight aortic stenosis or obstructive cardiomyopathy. Here exercise is often the precipitant.

Abnormalities of *heart rate and rhythm* may cause giddiness, faint feelings or LOC. About 20% of transient episodes of LOC are caused by disturbances of heart rate or rhythm. Usually the rate must be slow, less than 36/min, or fast, more than 180/min. Complete *heart block* may provoke *Stokes–Adams* attacks with sudden pallor and LOC from asystole lasting 5–12 seconds. As the circulation restores, the patient flushes. Such episodes may occur frequently. *Fast rates* often associated with palpitations may be due to a supraventricular tachycardia and these can lead to giddiness, and collapse with LOC. Sometimes these are triggered by exertion and may be followed by polyuria. A *sick sinus* (faulty 'ignition system') often from abnormal conduction in the sino-atrial node may cause a transient fall in cerebral perfusion.

Persistent abnormalities of rate and rhythm are easily recognised with the help of an ECG (electrocardiagram), but in patients with paroxysmal changes it may be necessary to refer them to hospital for ambulatory ECG monitoring with a portable continuous recording. It is important to instruct the patient to employ a marker button to demonstrate any periods when symptoms occur, as many patients with continuous recordings show asymptomatic changes of rate and rhythm.

Drugs can cause a fall in blood pressure. Ganglion blocking hypotensive agents are less commonly used but some dopa derivatives and vasodilators may cause a postural fall in blood pressure. A few Parkinsonian patients may already have a degree of autonomic upset so that dopa preparations may accentuate this.

Autonomic neuropathy is a rare cause of postural hypotension most often seen in diabetic patients with a neuropathy.

Transient hind brain ischaemia whether from migraine or vertebro-basilar disease may also cause transient LOC. In *basilar migraine* it is most common in teenage girls where there is commonly sufficient warning for them to lie down, becoming unrousable for 20–30 minutes. Severe occipital headache follows[6]. *Vertebro-basilar insufficiency* affects older patients, often women. Some show drop attacks falling to the ground without warning; often falling forward and sometimes sustaining injuries. Commonly there are other symptoms of brain stem upset – bilateral visual disturbances, diplopia, vertigo, circumoral tingling, alternating hemi-motor and sensory upsets, and speech slurring often with unsteadiness.

Vertebro-basilar ischaemic attacks in the elderly may arise from fibrin-platelet emboli, from disorders of blood flow (sometimes of cardiac origin) and sometimes on a mechanical basis where head turning may reduce flow in vertebral arteries already narrowed by atheroma. For treatment see Chapter 8.

Occasionally *acute vertigo* of labyrinthine origin may be accompanied by severe prostration with complaints of brief LOC.

TRANSIENT GLOBAL AMNESIA

This usually affects middle aged or elderly patients who suddenly develop episodes of complete amnesia often lasting several hours during which personal identity is retained but patients often repeatedly ask where they are and what they are doing. Observers will notice their behaviour seems abnormal. In some, the episodes seem precipitated by exercise, bathing in cold water or sexual intercourse. Some patients have isolated episodes, others repeated attacks. Most are thought due to vascular disease from transient ischaemia, but in a few an epileptic mechanism has been suggested.

EPILEPSY

This is a common disorder with an incidence in the U.K. of about 1 in 200 and some 250,000 patients on treatment. About 25,000 new patients will present each year. Thus a GP with an average list will have some 12–15 epileptic patients, half adults and half children.

A *seizure or fit* is produced by the sudden excessive disorderly discharge of brain cells. The term epilepsy is reserved for repeated seizures. The position, duration and site of this discharge influences the pattern of the attack. Many seizure classifications have been proposed but the table shows a simplification of the international scheme and divides seizures into those that are *generalised* from those with a focal or local origin, *partial* seizures. Partial seizures may spread and become generalised (Table 7). The importance of a partial seizure lies in the local site of origin where there may be an irritant focus from a scar or tumour[7]. In adult patients with cerebral tumours some 15–20% may have an epileptic seizure as the first symptom.

Serial major seizures or prolonged convulsing, lasting more than 30 minutes without recovery of consciousness is termed *status epilepticus*. This may be life-threatening and such patients need urgent measures to control their seizures and admission to hospital (see page 00).

Grand mal, major, tonic-clonic seizures

Here patients convulse. About a half have some warning, aura, but in the others there is sudden LOC. The aura may be an odd, slightly fearful sensation in the epigastric region, giddiness, or an involuntary twitch or jerk. These may herald the seizure. The patient then falls, is rigid in extension – the tonic phase. Some cry out. There is breath-holding, the eyes may open and stare or be deviated up or to one side. This may last 15–60 seconds and patients may become cyanosed. The clonic phase follows with involuntary jerking movements often accompanied by salivation, sometimes facial grimacing and eye rolling. There may be incontinence of urine, less commonly faeces. The clonic phase commonly last a few minutes and regular breathing does not start until there is relaxation from this.

Following this, patients then pass into a phase resembling sleep from which they cannot be easily roused. This usually lasts some minutes and during this there is usually no resistance to eye-opening and the plantar responses may be extensor. On recovery, patients are commonly confused, sleepy and often complain of headache. They may be aware then of a bitten tongue. A few vomit; many want to go back to sleep. Rarely the severity of the convulsion may provoke complaints of limb and backache, and even vertebral compression fractures from the force of the spasms.

Petit mal (absences)

These occur in children starting between the ages of 5–15 years and do not start in adults, although occasionally may persist from childhood into adult life. They consist of brief episodes, lasting 5–30 seconds, of loss of awareness during which the child stares. On recovery there is often blinking. There is no falling or involuntary limb movements.

The EEG (electroencephalogram) is characteristic with generalised three per second spike and wave discharges seen in most patients. Hyperventilation will provoke attacks in about 80%. Rarely serial absence seizures arise with the development of petit mal status, the affected child often appearing drowsy, unsteady, slowed and may dribble. There is impaired concentration in such episodes.

In some 85% of patients the attacks cease with increasing age but in a significant number they may be replaced by more major seizures.

Petit mal rarely arises *de novo* in adults.

Akinetic seizures, atonic, astatic attacks are uncommon but may arise in children where they are often associated with other types of seizures, particularly absences, tonic–clonic and myoclonic seizures. Many such children show evidence of brain damage with mental retardation and sometimes abnormal neurological signs. Such combinations of seizures often prove difficult to control.

Partial seizures

Simple partial seizures are best illustrated by the typical motor attack described by *Hughlings Jackson* where the site of onset lies in the motor cortex. This causes involuntary movements starting in the thumb, big toe or corner of the mouth. The movements usually spread or 'march' into the arm, leg and face involving the whole half of the body and limbs contralateral to the affected cortex. Sometimes the discharge will spread to produce a generalised seizure. Often there is no LOC and in some there may be turning of the head and eyes to the opposite side away from the irritated post-frontal area of the affected hemisphere (Figure 14a). Episodes last minutes and may be followed by transient limb weakness, a Todd's paresis, with an extensor plantar response. *Epilepsia partialis continua* describes continuous clonic twitching occurring in one group of muscles for prolonged periods of time. This is most often seen in the hand or foot.

Sensory seizures produce transient stereotyped episodes with tingling, numbness, brief shocks of pain, crawling sensations or even disordered body image. These are usually very brief and arise from the contralateral parietal area. The symptoms are most common in the face and arm, or the limbs and there again may be a 'march'.

Other sensory seizures may arise at other sites. Those from the occipital lobe may produce visual upset with colours, flashes, lights. Formed visual hallucinations arise from the temporal lobe.

Complex partial seizures

These usually have an *aura*, then a brief motor disturbance followed by a short period of confusion. There is LOC or loss of awareness, so patients are amnesic for the episode.

Many were originally described as temporal lobe epilepsy (TLE), sometimes as psychomotor seizures, as often the focus of origin was in the temporal lobe. However, a number may have an origin at other sites, e.g. the posterior part of the frontal lobe.

About two thirds of patients with complex partial seizures have a major seizure at some time.

The temporal lobes house memory, so auras include feelings of familiarity, *déjà vu*, or something that never happened, *jamais vu*. There may be formed hallucinations, visual or auditory, and olfactory and gustatory hallucinations – often an unpleasant smell or taste. Vertigo is a common aura. There may also be visceral symptoms with nausea and uneasiness. Speech upsets can occur in those with a dominant temporal lobe focus. Fear may also appear and even acute anxiety.

The *motor accompaniments* may be missed but include grimaces, lip smacking, teeth grinding, gulping, swallowing or chewing. Patients may grunt and stare. Sometimes they may move limbs – clench a hand, pluck at clothes, and even be incontinent.

More complex movements may follow an aura, *automatisms*, when patients perform actions, simple or complex, for which they have no recollection. Often they appear inappropriate when, for example a patient starts to undress on a bus, but they may lead to medico-legal problems as when patients are accused of shoplifting and claim no memory for the event. The diagnosis of epileptic automatisms is greatly aided for over 80% of such episodes are preceded by an aura, and in 80% the duration is less than five minutes.

Aggression is rare during an epileptic seizure. Patients may struggle if forcibly restrained. However, a proportion of teenagers with behaviour disorders may show EEG abnormalities and this may lead to the proposition that their anti-social behaviour or aggressive outbursts are epileptic. These are rarely so and it is more important to seek an eye-witnessed account and elicit any details of the attack than to rely on the EEG.

Table 8 Causes of epileptic seizures in adults

Idiopathic	Unknown. Usually start before the age of 20
Trauma	May follow perinatal injury or later head injury
Infection	Acutely with meningitis, encephalitis or cerebral abscess, or occur as a late complication
Vascular	Acutely with strokes or sub-arachnoid haemorrhage More common from the scar of a past infarct Also cortical thrombophlebitis, hypertensive encephalopathy
Tumours	Primary, benign or malignant Metastases
Metabolic	Hypoglycaemia, hypocalcaemia, uraemia, hepatic failure, porphyria, water intoxication
Drugs	INAH, tricyclic anti-depressants, lead poisoning Alcohol or barbiturate withdrawal
Degenerative	Alzheimer's disease, Jakob–Creutzfeldt's disease
Congenital	Tuberous sclerosis, neurofibromatosis

Causes of seizures are numerous; these are listed for adults in Table 8. In most young patients no obvious cause is found. In older patients over the age of 50 a vascular cause (scar from a stroke) is probably the commonest. In adults with late onset epilepsy some 10–15% are due to a cerebral tumour.

There is a *genetic* link although this is small. The risk of developing epilepsy is about 1 in 200. If one parent has epilepsy then the risk to the children of developing seizures is 1 in 40, if both parents have epilepsy then the risk rises to 1 in 4.

Most patients with epilepsy show *no* abnormal *signs*. A few show focal neurological abnormalities or signs of raised ICP. A few may also show skeletal asymmetries with perhaps mild underdevelopment of the limbs or face on one side which may indicate a long-standing fault with hemiatrophy of the opposite hemisphere. Rare cutaneous stigmata may be present as an angioma or adenoma sebaceum. There may sometimes be systemic abnormalities such as hypertension or an enlarged liver.

Triggers

Given sufficient provocation any patient may have an epileptic seizure and in some it appears the seizure threshold is low. Many triggers are recognised – high temperature, head injury, flashing lights, missed sleep, stress, menstrual periods. In a few patients seizures only occur at certain times, e.g. gestation or the withdrawal period after alcohol or barbiturate habituation. In some patients the avoidance of recognised triggers may reduce seizure frequency or prevent attacks.

Investigation

Certain tests can be arranged by GPs to look at causes and also sometimes to establish if episodes of LOC are epileptic. These should include:

(1) A blood sample for (a) full blood count and ESR
                        (b) blood glucose, calcium and urea
                        (c) WR or equivalent (VDRL, TPHA or FTA)

(2) X-rays of the chest and skull.

Most adults developing epileptic seizures should be referred to a physician or neurologist. At the hospital they will usually have an EEG and CT brain scan. An ECG may be helpful if there is a possible circulatory factor.

All patients with *focal symptoms* and *signs* or those with features of *raised ICP* require hospital referral.

A normal EEG does not exclude the diagnosis of epilepsy and conversely an abnormal EEG does not mean the patient must have seizures. Some 10–15% of the 'normal population' who have never had a seizure may show an abnormal EEG. However, an EEG may show a clear discharging focus or a slow wave abnormality and these may indicate the need for further investigation.

More detailed studies and even in-patient observation may be necessary if there is diagnostic doubt or very frequent seizures. The most sophisticated units rely on closed circuit TV monitoring with continuous EEG telemetry.

Treatment

It is important to instruct relatives about how to cope with a patient having a major seizure. The best position is lying semi-prone with a cushion or pillow under the hips so the bottom is higher than the head, which allows any secretions to run out of the mouth, aided by gravity. Serial major seizures or continuous convulsions may indicate an incipient status epilepticus which is an emergency (page 54).

It is not usual to treat an isolated seizure but patients who have had two or more seizures in a relatively short time need anticonvulsant drugs (ACs) to control further attacks. In a few high risk situations prophylactic ACs may be used – e.g. after a penetrating head injury or brain abscess.

47

There are many ACs, and GPs are advised to learn a few, in particular their dose range, indications, half-life, side effects and efficacy in certain types of seizure (Tables 9 and 10).

Grand mal seizures are most easily controlled. Complex partial seizures are the most difficult. In about four fifths of patients good control with ACs can be obtained.

Start with a *single appropriate AC* in the usual adult dose and follow progress. If seizures continue then the *serum AC level* can be measured but sufficient time must have elapsed to give a steady level. This depends on the drug's half-life and phenytoin or phenobarbitone may take seven to ten days to reach a steady state. If the level is low then the dose may be increased, unless compliance is suspect. However, it should be emphasised that in some patients with good seizure control there may be a low blood level (sub-therapeutic). If frequent seizures persist despite a therapeutic drug level then either a different drug should be substituted, adding the new AC before slowly tapering off the old one, or the seizures should be reassessed. What is the cause? Could these be non-epileptic seizures? An AC should not be stopped suddenly as this may precipitate seizures or even status.

In a small group of patients seizures are *difficult to control*. This may reflect the cause for their seizures, e.g. widespread brain damage. Here polypharmacy is common. In such patients the use

Table 9 Drugs used in the treatment of epileptic seizures

Grand mal, tonic–clonic	1. phenytoin
	2. carbamazepine
	3. valproate sodium
	4. phenobarbitone, primidone
Petit mal, absences	1. valproate sodium
	2. ethosuximide
Partial – simple, complex	1. carbamazepine
	2. phenytoin
Myoclonic, akinetic	1. valproate sodium
	2. clonazepam

The numbers indicate the authors' preference in these seizure types

Table 10 Anticonvulsant drugs

| Drug | Dose range | | Half-life hours | Levels | |
	Children mg/kg/day	Adults mg/day		µg/ml	µmol/l
Carbamazepine (Tegretol)	10 – 20	600 – 1,200	12 – 40	3 – 10	13 – 42
Ethosuximide (Zarontin)	20 – 30	750 – 1,000	30 – 60	40 – 120	280 – 840
Phenobarbitone (Gardenal, Luminal)	3 – 5	60 – 180	80 – 120	15 – 40	60 – 176
Phenytoin (Epanutin)	4 – 7	300 – 400	24 – 36	10 – 20	40 – 80
Primidone* (Mysoline)	10 – 25	750 – 1,000	12 – 18	5 – 15	23 – 69
Valproate sodium	20 – 30	1,000 – 2,400	6 – 12	30 – 100	210 – 700

*Primidone is broken down into phenobarbitone and phenylethylmalonamide
Most drugs reach a 'steady state' within one to two weeks of treatment – about four times the half-life

of two or three ACs gives rise to a higher incidence of side effects. Toxic drug levels of phenytoin may actually cause more frequent seizures.

In well-controlled epileptic patients taking two or three ACs, it may prove unwise to try and reduce their medication as this may provoke further seizures; important if they have regained their driving licence.

Combinations of ACs often cause competition in liver pathways and this will produce changes in the drug levels of each drug. This may lead to poor seizure control or the production of toxic effects. Other drugs may also interfere, for example a low dose oestrogen-containing *contraceptive pill* will compete with phenytoin or carbamazepine lowering their blood levels. Sometimes this may aggravate seizure control. Conversely these two ACs make the 'pill' less effective as a contraceptive. Valproate is the only AC that does not compete with the 'pill'.

Side effects

All ACs may produce *toxic dose-related side effects* particularly ataxia, drowsiness, slurred speech, diplopia and disturbed cognitive function (i.e. like a 'drunk'). Reduction in the dose will reduce such effects. In a few sensitive patients allergic skin rashes may arise. Rarely, long term use of ACs may cause problems as osteomalacia.

Phenytoin has a narrow therapeutic range so a small dose increase may produce toxic blood levels. Phenytoin may also produce gum hypertrophy, hirsutism, aggravate acne, and occasionally cause lymph gland enlargement and macrocytic anaemia. Very rarely it may cause cerebellar damage, chorea and a peripheral neuropathy.

Phenobarbitone should be avoided in the young and the elderly. It is likely to cause depression and drowsiness. In the young it may also produce overactivity and even aggression and adversely affect learning. In the elderly, confusion may be a problem. *Primidone* is largely broken down into phenobarbitone and phenylethyl-malonamide. It has the same barbiturate side effects. In a propor-tion of patients starting primidone treatment an acute cerebellar syndrome arises (vomiting, unsteadiness). This usually can be prevented by the slow introduction of the drug and then increasing the dose in small increments.

Carbamazepine is particularly useful in complex partial seizures and in major seizures in adolescent girls and young women. Rarely it may cause drug rashes (some 3%), liver damage and very occa-sionally marrow depression.

Valproate may cause weight gain, hair thinning, tremor and very rarely liver damage which in a few patients has proved fatal. However, such reports all seem to have occurred within six months of starting treatment often in already neurologically 'damaged' children. Obviously valproate should be avoided in patients with a history of liver damage or abnormal liver function tests. Valproate has the advantage of being effective in the control of petit mal and grand mal.

Ethosuximide is only useful in the treatment of petit mal. It does not help to control other types of seizure. The side effects are drowsiness, headache, gastrointestinal upsets and, rarely, rashes and leucopenia.

Clonazepam is at present the most effective of the oral ben-zodiazepines in controlling epileptic seizures. It is useful in petit mal, myoclonic attacks and major seizures. It may cause drowsi-ness and unsteadiness. In children irritability and increased saliva-tion may also occur.

All ACs may have a small *teratogenic risk*. However, this needs to be balanced against the real risks to mother and foetus from uncontrolled major seizures. Furthermore, in most epileptic patients, by the time pregnancy is confirmed, they are usually eight to ten weeks pregnant. Most epileptic mothers need to continue their drugs through pregnancy. It is probably wise to give generous folic acid supplements as well. If a woman has been seizure-free for some time (two or more years) and is planning a pregnancy, then ideally the ACs should be tapered off first.

ACs will pass into *breast milk* but only in small amounts which a baby will excrete, so epileptic mothers on treatment can breast-feed.

Driving and epilepsy

It is a doctor's duty to tell patients the law about driving. The onus is on the patient to declare any relevant disability lasting more than three months to the DVLC (Driver Vehicle Licensing Centre) at Swansea. The doctor must tell them if they have such disability. Patients who ignore cautions that they are ineligible may find their insurance cover is void and they can be prosecuted. If a doctor has not told a patient they are ineligible then that doctor may share part of the responsibility for any accident that might follow.

Any patient who has had two or more epileptic seizures is not entitled to drive until they have been two or more years seizure-free. Petit mal, simple and complex partial seizures are included. Patients who are seizure-free for more than two years and are still taking ACs may drive providing they continue with their therapy. If they are tapering off their drugs or significantly altering the dose, they should not drive and a period of at least six months should elapse before driving is resumed to check there is no seizure recurrence.

Patients who only have had seizures in sleep for more than three years may drive on the assumption that it is then unlikely that they will develop diurnal fits. However, this is a very small group.

In patients where there has been only a single seizure, the rules are less clear. Most doctors and the DVLC interpret these by suggesting that if no cause is found then a ban for twelve months should be imposed. If, however, an obvious cause is present, e.g. the scar from an infarct or an irritable EEG focus, then a two year ban is necessary.

Any patient who has had an epileptic seizure after the age of five is precluded from an HGV (Heavy Goods Vehicle) or PSV (Public Service Vehicle) licence.

It is always possible for doctors to write to the DVLC to ask for advice about any driving problem; a ruling will then be given.

Epilepsy and employment

Certain occupations are barred to patients with epilepsy. These include the armed forces, the police, holders of HGV or PSV licences, or air-line pilots.

Epileptic patients should also be advised not to seek a job where their employment relies on driving. They should also avoid occupations where working at heights or over-exposed machinery parts might give increased risks of injury.

Large firms employ doctors who will give advice to the firm about the suitability of a patient to certain tasks in the context of the firm's responsibility for industrial injuries sustained while at work.

Unfortunately, there is still a stigma attached to the label of epilepsy and occasionally a single seizure at work is used as excuse for dismissal. However, in the majority of patients with reasonable seizure control, employment is possible. A few patients, either because of the severity or frequency of their seizures, or because of the underlying disease causing them, may be unemployable or even need institutional care.

A patient with epilepsy can be registered as disabled and be eligible for retraining. They may also then have the help of the DRO in seeking work.

Duration of treatment

In a proportion of children or adolescents who develop epileptic seizures, with increasing time the seizures cease and it may be possible to taper off the ACs. However, in adults with later onset fits, the chances are much less. Recent studies have suggested in adults who present with a single seizure over one third will have further attacks over the next two years; most in the first twelve months[8].

In patients who have gone three years seizure-free probably about one third will have further fits if the ACs are discontinued. Obviously, a significant cerebral scar, irritant EEG focus or underlying persistent brain disease leaves a higher recurrence risk. Many such patients may be safer continuing ACs indefinitely. In patients whose seizures start after the age of 50 and persist, there is probably only a 50% chance of the seizures stopping. However, the longer patients go seizure-free the better is the chance that they may be able to discontinue treatment. Medication should always be tapered off slowly.

It should be remembered that adults who have gone two years seizure-free, with attacks controlled by ACs, often are not prepared to stop driving. While stopping treatment they temporarily will have to cease driving, and for some months afterwards.

Status epilepticus

This is a *medical emergency*. Either there is continuous convulsing or serial tonic–clonic seizures without recovery of consciousness lasting more than 30 minutes. In both states, unchecked seizures may cause anoxia with hyperpyrexia, sometimes irreversible brain damage and even death.

Most bouts of status arise in known epileptics with poor seizure control although occasional patients present in status. In such patients a proportion may show evidence of a frontal tumour. In some patients status may be precipitated by the sudden cessation of AC therapy, an infection or injury.

The GP faced with such a patient must:

(1) Try and *prevent any respiratory obstruction*. The patient should be positioned head down, semi-prone, preferably with an airway inserted into the mouth.

(2) Try and *stop the seizures* while an ambulance is called and the patient is transferred to hospital. Most patients will respond

to intravenous (IV) diazepam given slowly. Adults require 10 mg, children 0.3 mg/kg or 1 mg per year of life. Diazemuls has a very much lower incidence of phlebitis. Diazepam may prove to have a rather short duration of action and the authors prefer IV clonazepam (Rivotril). Adults require 1 mg, children about 0.5 mg, IV given slowly; this is more effective and longer lasting.

If there is likely to be delay before transfer, the above measures should be followed by the setting up of an IV infusion preferably in a vein away from any joint where convulsive movements might dislodge the needle. This will allow access for any further drugs.

In some patients there may be difficulty in finding a vein. Here *rectal diazepam* may be used. Diazepam is rapidly absorbed from the lining of the rectum within a few minutes (4–10 minutes). In adults the dose is 10 mg, in children less than three years old 0.2 mg/kg. The Stesolid disposable rectal dispenser is most useful: this will give a 5 or 10 mg dose. An intramuscular (IM) injection of paraldehyde, in adults 5–10 ml, in children 0.15 ml/kg, may sometimes be used but the injections are painful and are certainly a second choice.

Febrile convulsions

These are common in children between the ages of six months and six years: about 4% of all children will convulse with a high temperature. The attack is usually brief, lasting less than 10 minutes and the child makes a full recovery. The EEG is normal between attacks. However, some 10–15% probably go on to develop epilepsy; furthermore there is evidence to suggest that prolonged febrile convulsions may lead to hippocampal damage (Ammon's horn sclerosis) which may then act as a focus for the continuation of complex partial seizures in adult life.

This has led to the proposal that children at risk should be given prophylactic ACs. However, this treatment in young children has caused problems (particularly with phenobarbitone) and all trials have shown a significant number who stop treatment because of side effects.

Do you *admit all children* suspected of a first febrile convulsion? The answer is yes. It is safer to admit any child with a first febrile convulsion; for children with meningitis may present with a convulsion and a temperature. Very young children may show no meningism. Furthermore, a convulsion is a frightening experience and one recent survey showed 60% of such children were immediately sent by their parents to hospital[9].

In older children (over the age of two) with a past history of febrile convulsions (one third have repeated attacks), who are seen at a time when they have recovered, have an obvious infective source and responsible parents, it may be possible to nurse these at home. Febrile convulsions are very rare starting *de novo* after the age of five. Children with prolonged or repeated attacks, post-ictal focal signs or an unexplained high temperature will need admission.

If a child has had a febrile convulsion, parents should be advised how to treat any fever by cooling, tepid sponging if necessary, and the use of paracetamol (Calpol) or aspirin. It is also possible to give rectal diazepam to children who have a high temperature as a prophylactic measure.

In the *high risk patients*, phenobarbitone and valproate (not phenytoin or carbamazepine) have both been shown to be effective in preventing further attacks. The high risk group includes children with any prolonged generalised or focal attack (more than 30 minutes), repeated seizures, with signs of previous neurological damage or signs after an attack, and those whose attacks start before the age of 18 months. Most of these children are referred to hospital clinics.

Childhood seizures

The GP is less likely to be involved with *neonatal seizures* in the first few days of life, but it should be remembered that in the first

14 days these may arise from brain damage, either from a difficult birth or anoxia, or from hypoglycaemia. Less commonly hypocalcaemia, pyridoxine deficiency, hypomagnesaemia and rare inborn errors of metabolism may be responsible. Brain damage is more likely to produce tonic seizures, whereas metabolic upsets are more likely to cause clonic seizures.

At all ages *meningitis* may present with seizures and in the very young, the very old or the very ill there may be no meningism. Seizures may also follow head injury, metabolic disturbances or even be precipitated by breath-holding. Petit mal presents in childhood.

Childhood-onset seizures with a worse outlook are *infantile spasms or salaam attacks*. These start between the ages of 3–9 months. Many of the children show evidence of brain damage with features of mental retardation which may reflect pre-, peri- or post-natal damage. The attacks are often repeated with the baby flexing forward from the waist in a salaam and drawing up their legs. The EEG may show a characteristic disturbance. In some children steroids as well as ACs may help control attacks. Any form of epileptic seizure in an infant (one year or less) requires referral to a paediatrician.

Some children may have prolonged focal convulsing followed by a residual *hemiparesis*. Occasionally this may persist and then be followed by failure of full development in the hemiparetic limbs, i.e. an infantile hemiplegia. Such patients often show a hemiatrophy of the affected hemisphere which may lead to persistent seizures.

Myoclonus is a sudden involuntary jerk, usually of the arms (page 164). This may herald a major seizure or occur in certain metabolic upsets, e.g. uraemia, or after anoxia. Myoclonus may also occur in rare encephalitic processes as sub-acute sclerosing panencephalitis or CNS degenerative conditions as gangliosidoses. These are usually accompanied by mental retardation and major seizures. Clonazepam may help control myoclonus. Children with repeated seizures, bizarre attacks, any suggestion of mental retardation or failure to develop, or the presence of abnormal neurological signs will be referred to hospital.

Childhood seizures will necessitate considerable *explanation* and *support* for the family with the need for advice about how to manage the seizure, what restrictions to impose, the need to control attacks with ACs, and how best for the child to achieve at school. Most children are able to attend normal schools and take part in sporting activities. Rock climbing, unsupervised swimming and bicycling on crowded roads should be avoided.

BREATH-HOLDING ATTACKS

These may appear in children aged nine months to six years. They are often triggered by fear or pain, sometimes frustration or anger and the child seems to cry soundlessly holding their breath. This causes loss of consciousness, cyanosis, stiffening and even a convulsion. The attacks are brief and the child appears to recover rapidly. In a second 'pallid form', there is no crying and the child collapses limply with temporary circulatory arrest. In this group ocular compression may cause temporary asystole.

Children are normal between attacks; the EEG is normal and the attacks are self-limiting. Parents will need reassurance and advice about management.

NARCOLEPSY

This is characterised by excessive day-time sleepiness often accompanied by disturbed night-time sleep. Gélineau's syndrome describes a combination of narcolepsy, cataplexy (transient sudden falling usually provoked by emotion), sleep paralysis (transient total immobility on waking or falling asleep), and hypnagogic hallucinations (vivid visual hallucinations in sleep).

In normal sleep periods of relative light sleep, REM (rapid eye movement) are interspersed with deeper sleep (non-REM). This pattern is disturbed in the narcoleptic. Attacks usually start in adolescence or early adult life and tend to persist. There is a positive family history in about 25%.

Most patients have just the sleep episodes usually lasting about ten minutes but repeated several times daily. The attacks may occur at odd times such as during eating or even driving and in such situations may suggest the diagnosis. Thus narcoleptics should not drive.

Rarely excessive sleepiness may occur with brain tumours – particularly hypothalamic, or in encephalitis, or more commonly with drug abuse.

Treatment of narcolepsy is with amphetamine-like substances. Unfortunately, these are all addicting and as sympathomimetic amines may elevate blood pressure. Methylphenidate (Ritalin) 20–60 mg daily is most commonly used starting with the smallest effective dose. Clomipramine (Anafranil) 10–25 mg nocte is very useful in cataplexy and sleep paralysis.

HYPOGLYCAEMIA

This most often follows missing food or insulin overdosage in treated diabetics but may occur with rare insulinomas or even in alcoholic liver disease. With blood glucose levels of less than 2.2 mmol/l (40 mg/%) there are usually warning symptoms with confusion, irritability, slurred speech, weakness (which may even be focal) and ataxia. Sometimes patients are mistakenly thought to be drunk. Later patients become stuporose, unconscious and if prolonged coma follows, irreversible brain damage may occur. Hypoglycaemia also provokes adrenaline release with pallor, sweating (a cold moist skin), apprehension, headache and even tingling.

If the diagnosis is suspected, a blood sample for a glucose level should be taken and the patient immediately given glucose, preferably IV.

HYPOCALCAEMIA

This is rare and usually follows parathyroid removal after surgery, often of the thyroid, or from primary failure of the parathyroid gland or severe malabsorption. A low calcium level (less than 2.2 mmol/l) will cause neuromuscular irritability with the development of tetany, numbness and tingling around the mouth and in the extremities, and even carpopedal spasms (sometimes mistaken for tonic seizures). Muscles may appear weak with a proximal myopathy but the reflexes are exaggerated. Patients may also develop cataracts and swelling of the optic discs. There may also be mental changes with anxiety, depression and sometimes changes in the skin and nails.

Hypoglycaemia and hypocalcaemia may trigger epileptic seizures.

Hyperventilation in anxious patients will provoke a respiratory alkalosis with tingling around the mouth and in the extremities. These are often accompanied by light headed, giddy and faint feelings with a sensation of breathlessness. If over-breathing continues then muscle twitching, carpopedal spasm and even LOC may follow. Attacks may last 10–30 minutes. In patients suspected of hyperventilation a trial of over-breathing for three minutes will usually reproduce the symptoms.

Benign cryptogenic drop attacks arise in middle aged women[10]. They cause sudden episodes of falling, usually forward onto the knees. Sometimes patients sustain injuries but they do not lose consciousness. The cause is uncertain. They do not respond to anti-convulsants nor to anti-coagulants. In many patients they disappear with time.

Non-epileptic seizures These are fairly common and difficult to diagnose. They are most frequent in girls and young women who may show an appropriate background history of disturbed behaviour and emotions. Some patients have obvious gain from such attacks which occur before an audience. Relatives, nursing staff and doctors may recognise the nature of the attacks.

Table 11 Differential diagnosis of epileptic from hysterical seizures

	Epileptic	*Hysterical, non-epileptic*
Cause	absent	emotional upset
Warning	50% aura, 50% none	varied, palpitations, malaise
Onset	sudden	gradual
Motor	tonic then clonic	struggling proportional to restraint, bizarre postures
Biting	tongue frequent	lips, hands, other people
Eyelids	easy to open, may be open with eyes deviated	eyelids difficult to open
Incontinence	frequent	never
Plantars	often extensor	flexor
Duration	minutes usually	often prolonged
Sequel	confused, drowsy	exhausted, 'drained'

Adapted from Gowers (1885)[11]

The guide-lines suggested by Gowers[11] are still valid (Table 11). Attacks tend to have a slow build-up. Struggling is often proportional to the degree of restraint used and there is seldom incontinence or tongue biting. In the attack it may be difficult to open the eyes due to volitional eyelid closure and the plantar responses do not become extensor.

There may be difficulty in establishing the mechanism in some patients, particularly in those who also have genuine epileptic seizures. Suspicion may be aroused in patients who continue to have frequent bizarre attacks in the presence of therapeutic blood levels of a main-line anti-convulsant. Here in-patient observation may be necessary to elucidate the problem.

A therapeutic trial with ACs is not a good approach. If there is doubt about the diagnosis it is better to await events observing the attacks. True seizures will become apparent.

If the diagnosis is unclear with regard to episodes of loss of consciousness or awareness, it is better to admit uncertainty than mislabel a patient as 'epileptic', particularly if the episodes are functional.

4

Giddiness

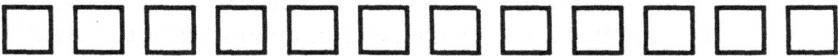

DEFINITION

Giddiness, dizziness, vertigo are difficult symptoms to assess. In many instances the patient's understanding is different to that of the doctor. Vertigo is a hallucination of movement, either of the patient or their surrounds. Acute vertigo is commonly associated with nausea, vomiting, pallor, perspiration, prostration and a sense of fear. These are well illustrated in acute motion sickness. In assessing giddiness it is important to ask if the symptoms arise in the head, are intermittent or persistent, and if there are any associated features or positional triggers. Rather non-specific complaints of faint or light headed feelings, particularly of long duration, are usually benign and often functional.

ANATOMY

The balance apparatus includes the two organs of balance, the vestibular nerves and their central connexions in the brain stem. These are intimately linked with the cerebellum. The visual system, position sense in the limbs, neck reflexes and higher cortical centres also add their influence.

SIGNS

Disturbance of the balance mechanism may produce nystagmus and ataxy of stance and gait. Sometimes there is limb incoordination and dysarthria, particularly if there is cerebellar upset. Many peripheral disorders of balance show a change of *hearing*. This may be tested by audiometry. Auditory evoked potentials may be used to measure conduction in the brain stem. *Caloric tests* use irrigation of the external auditory canals with hot and cold water, to provoke convection currents in the semi-circular canals and so produce nystagmus through an oculo-vestibular reflex. These test vestibular function which may also be tested by electro-nystagmography (ENG). The pathway involves the semi-circular canals, the eighth cranial nerve, and pontine pathways extending up to the level of the oculomotor nuclei.

NYSTAGMUS

Jerk nystagmus from *peripheral vestibular damage* (in the labyrinth) arises with the fast phase (direction of the nystagmus) directed away from the side of damage. This nystagmus is horizontal, unidirectional and enhanced by loss of fixation such as eye closure, darkness or the use of Frenzel's lenses (high plus lenses which defocus the eyes).

Central vestibular damage in the brain stem or cerebellum (and connections) will produce a more coarse nystagmus, usually ipsilateral towards the side of the lesion. It is sometimes bidirectional (to either side) and even vertical or rotatory. This is often inhibited by darkness or eye closure. Such central damage is commonly associated with the presence of abnormal cerebellar signs.

ACUTE VERTIGO

This may arise as a single severe episode or in repeated attacks. The latter are most commonly due to a peripheral labyrinthine disturbance.

Acute labyrinthine failure may arise in several ways: from *infection* as in purulent middle ear infection where there is often aural discharge. *All* patients should have their *ears examined*. A less common infective cause is *herpes zoster* which is often accompanied by a lower motor neurone facial weakness. Herpetic vesicles may be visible in the external ear.

Head injuries, including 'whip lash' injuries to the neck, may also cause acute vertigo with often positional aggravation. *Acute poisoning* with alcohol or salicylates may cause vertigo. Bilateral labyrinthine or vestibular nerve damage may follow the use of certain *ototoxic drugs*, e.g. gentamicin, quinine. This is more common in elderly patients with renal damage and may prove irreversible. Surgical destruction of one labyrinth will cause vertigo, vomiting and imbalance usually settling in two to three weeks.

ACUTE VESTIBULAR FAILURE

This may arise in young adults labelled as an acute labyrinthitis or vestibular neuronitis. A viral aetiology is often presumed. Patients present with prostrating vertigo and vomiting confining them to bed. They usually lie supine, avoiding position changes which aggravate their symptoms. Such patients may show fine horizontal nystagmus (away from the affected ear) and unsteadiness. There is an absent caloric response on the affected side. Hearing is spared. The attack is usually self-limiting over some two or three weeks but many patients show residual imbalance with positional giddiness for some weeks after the acute attack.

Treatment

This is symptomatic with initial bed rest, anti-emetics and vestibular sedatives. Prochlorperazine (Stemetil) 5–10 mg t.i.d. as tablets, or the use of suppositories (25 mg in adults), or even 12.5 mg by injection may prove helpful. Occasionally young adults, often women, may develop an acute dystonic reaction to phenothiazines, such as tonic deviation of the eyes.

BENIGN POSITIONAL VERTIGO

Here recurrent brief attacks of vertigo arise which are triggered by a change of position – most often on lying down or sitting up, but occasionally with head turning or bending. Such episodes arise from the otolith in the utricle and may follow head injury, infection or be of unknown cause. The diagnosis can be confirmed in the surgery or at the bedside by eliciting positional nystagmus. Patients are tested sitting (Figure 6) with the head turned to one side. They are asked to stare at the examiner's nose and then are rapidly laid flat with the head still slightly turned but now a little lower than the trunk. Susceptible patients show acute vertigo (which makes them want to shut their eyes) after a latent interval of a few seconds with a rotatory coarse nystagmus towards the undermost ear (the affected otolith). The nystagmus and vertigo settle within 10–20 seconds but may be repeated as the patient sits up. Repeated testing shows the vertigo and nystagmus to fatigue (disappear). Only one side is affected.

The condition is self-limiting but reassurance and the use of vestibular sedatives (cinnarizine (Stugeron) or prochlorperazine) and head-turning exercises may be beneficial.

Central brain stem lesions rarely may cause positional vertigo and nystagmus. This nystagmus has no latent interval, persists, does not fatigue and does not reverse direction from sitting to lying and vice versa.

OTHER RECURRENT CAUSES OF VERTIGO

These include *transient brain stem ischaemia*. This may arise in young patients as the build-up to a migraine attack (page 21) where the vertigo is followed by severe headache and vomiting which may aid diagnosis. In older patients, episodic vertigo from

Figure 6 Testing for positional nystagmus and vertigo

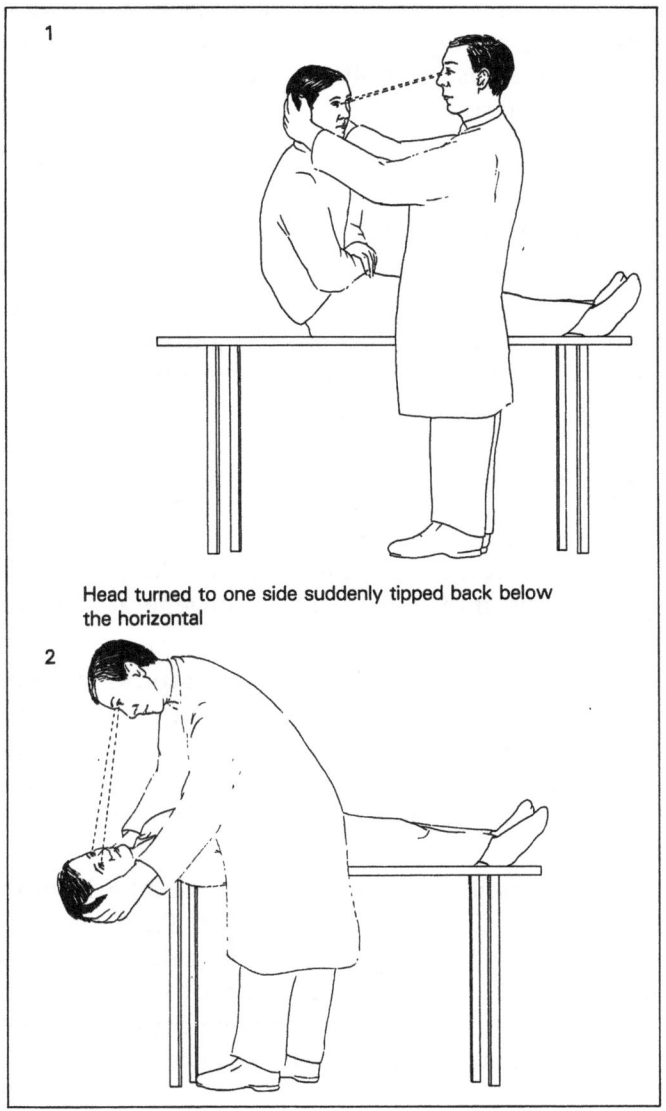

Head turned to one side suddenly tipped back below the horizontal

brain stem ischaemia may arise from vertebro-basilar insufficiency but in such patients there are often symptoms of visual, speech or limb disturbance as well as other pointers to vascular disease. Giddiness may be a symptom of a drop in cerebral perfusion, e.g. heart block, sick sinus (page 40) or even the prodrome of some epileptic seizures (page 44).

BENIGN PAROXYSMAL VERTIGO

This arises in children between the ages of three and eight. It causes recurrent attacks. These prove self-limiting and often require no treatment once they are recognised. Caloric tests will show a canal paresis of the affected labyrinth.

MÉNIÈRE'S DISEASE

In older patients this is the main cause of recurrent episodes of vertigo lasting more than a minute or two. Ménière's disease is possibly a hydrops of the labyrinth with degeneration of the cochlear hair cells.

Patients complain of more protracted attacks of prostrating vertigo usually lasting minutes to hours and accompanied by vomiting. There is commonly some deafness, often tinnitus and in the attack these may appear more severe, often associated with a feeling of fullness in the affected ear. Many patients are intolerant of a loud noise.

In the attacks patients appear unsteady with horizontal nystagmus directed away from the affected ear. They have a sensori-neural deafness with loudness recruitment (selective destruction of the low intensity elements in the organ of Corti) and impaired caloric tests on the affected side. With an acoustic neuroma there may be sensori-neural deafness with absence of loudness recruitment (page 71).

With repeated attacks there is often increasing deafness and this may be accompanied by significant anxiety. In nearly one third of patients the disease becomes bilateral.

Treatment

The response is variable. In acute attacks bed rest is important. Most patients find benefit from vestibular sedatives – betahistine (Serc) 8 mg t.i.d. cinnarizine (Stugeron) 15–30 mg t.i.d., or anti-histamines as diphenhydramine hydrochloride (Benadryl) 25–50 mg t.i.d. or dimenhydrinate (Dramamine) 50–100 mg repeated after four hours in an attack.

In severely affected patients with failure of medical treatment, surgical measures may be helpful. Endolymph sac drainage may relieve vertigo without affecting hearing in about two thirds of patients. If patients have significant deafness the destruction of the affected labyrinth may give relief (this will destroy any residual hearing on the affected side).

CENTRAL CAUSES OF ACUTE PERSISTING VERTIGO

Acute episodes of vertigo of rather longer duration may follow damage to the central connexions in the brain stem. In younger patients this may be due to a plaque of *demyelination* (multiple sclerosis – MS) and in older patients, a *stroke*. In the former, patients may give a past history of other episodes of central nervous system disturbance. In the latter, there may be features to suggest widespread vascular disease (hypertension, previous myocardial damage).

Signs and symptoms

Such attacks arise acutely with vertigo, vomiting, unsteadiness and often slurred speech. Hearing is usually spared but patients often complain of visual upset (diplopia or blurring), hiccup, difficulties swallowing and sensory upsets which may involve the face and limbs. Often such patients show coarse nystagmus, multidirectional or vertical, disordered conjugate eye movements, a Horner's syndrome (ipsilateral to the site of damage) and also ipsilateral cerebellar signs in the limbs. There is ataxy of stance and gait which is very prominent if mid-line cerebellar structures are damaged. The lower cranial nerves may sometimes be involved with facial and bulbar weakness. Pyramidal signs may appear in the limbs. Spinothalamic sensory loss may occur in the face on one side and this may be accompanied by a similar pattern sensory upset in the limbs and trunk either on the same side as the face or on the opposite side depending on the level of the brain stem damage.

Symptoms and signs usually persist for days, sometimes weeks, particularly if there has been a brain stem infarct, but often there is slow improvement. Most patients require referral to hospital and often admission. Bed rest, anti-emetics and sedatives may give symptomatic relief. In known MS patients a short course of steroids may dramatically relieve an acute brain stem plaque.

PERSISTENT UNSTEADINESS – ATAXIA

Anatomy

This most often arises from the cerebellum and central vestibular pathways in the brain stem, but may also follow severe peripheral labyrinthine damage (e.g. from gentamicin), severe posterior column damage (e.g tabes dorsalis), and hydrocephalus (obstructive and normal pressure). It may also be found with postural disturbance in Parkinson's disease and in patients with a high cervical cord lesion (damaging the posterior columns above C 3/4). In the last there is loss of position sense in the fingers often accompanied by pseudo-athetosis (involuntary 'piano-playing' finger movements best seen in the out-stretched hands). All forms of sensory ataxia are worsened by eye closure and patients show Rombergism (increased unsteadiness with eye closure) and usually absent limb reflexes.

Cerebellar signs

Lateralised cerebellar damage causes incoordination of the ipsilateral limbs with intention tremor. This may be accompanied by dysarthria, nystagmus, and unsteadiness of stance and gait with a tendency to fall to the affected side if the patient walks around a chair. There is difficulty hopping on the ipsilateral foot in mildly affected patients. Tandem stance and walking heel–toe along a line will show mild disorders of mid-line cerebellar damage (the vermis).

Cerebellopontine angle tumours

The most common tumour here is an *acoustic neuroma* arising on the eighth cranial nerve. This is slow growing and as it expands in the internal auditory canal (porus) it causes *progressive deafness*, and impaired balance from compression of the cochlear and vestibular divisions. The deafness is sensori-neural in type with absence of loudness recruitment. Caloric tests are abnormal and AEPs are also disturbed. X-rays of the petrous bones may show widening of the porus in 70–80%.

Signs and symptoms

In addition to eighth nerve involvement, other cranial nerves may be compressed in the order of:

(1) Trigeminal.
(2) Abducens.
(3) Facial.
(4) Bulbar (cranial nerves 10 and 12).

About one quarter of patients show a neuroma expanding medially and compressing the brain stem at a relatively early stage. This may cause coarse nystagmus, ataxy, headache with features of raised intracranial pressure (from an obstructive hydrocephalus) as well as deafness.

An acoustic neuroma may be part of generalised neurofibromatosis. Other angle tumours include a meningioma, metastasis, cholesteatoma and aneurysm.

Patients suspected of having an acoustic neuroma require hospital referral. Early diagnosis is important for complete removal with preservation of the facial nerve, and this may be possible if the tumour is small. With large tumours there is an appreciable morbidity and mortality.

PROGRESSIVE UNSTEADINESS

Here patients require referral to hospital. In all patients, hearing and balance should be tested. In children there is a high incidence of posterior fossa tumours (medulloblastomas, cerebellar astrocytomas, and ependymomas)[12]. In most patients CT scanning is necessary to see if there is any evidence of a posterior fossa tumour. In some patients this may be extrinsic and surgically removable.

In older patients, infarcts, degenerative conditions and hydrocephalus need consideration. In younger patients the presence of scoliosis, pes cavus, diabetes mellitus or any family history of unsteadiness raises the question of a spinocerebellar degeneration (e.g. Friedreich's ataxia, page 149).

Family doctors should arrange:

(1) A blood sample to exclude polycythaemia or myxoedema.

(2) A chest X-ray to exclude the presence of a lung cancer which either may have metastasised to the posterior fossa or rarely produced a non-metastatic cerebellar degeneration.

(3) Plain X-rays of the skull with views of the internal auditory canals. These may show features of raised intracranial pressure or an expanded porus. Children with posterior fossa masses often show signs of raised intracranial pressure with radiological changes on the skull X-rays.

In the *very old patient* unsteadiness is common. The causes are often multiple (page 159).

Vestibular sedatives are disappointing in patients with unsteadiness of central origin or cerebellar damage. Drug treatment of cerebellar symptoms is not at present effective. *Balancing exercises* given by physiotherapists may help some patients.

5

Facial Pain

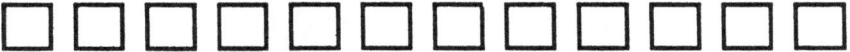

ANATOMY

The trigeminal nerve supplies the face (Figure 7). It has its sensory nuclei in the pons. The chief nucleus lies in the tegmentum and relays touch. The descending spinal nucleus passes into the upper cervical cord, as low as C 2, and relays pain and temperature. There is also a high mesencephalic nucleus at the level of the colliculi concerned with proprioception. The trigeminal nerve splits into three main divisions at the Gasserian ganglion which is sited at the petrous apex in the middle cranial fossa (Figure 8).

The *ophthalmic division* supplies the frontal region, top of the scalp as far back as the lambdoid suture (Figure 7), the eye ball, orbit and linings of much of the nose. The branch passes through the orbit entering the skull via the superior orbital fissure, and then passing through the cavernous sinus goes to join the ganglion. In the cavernous sinus it lies close to the oculomotor and abducens nerves and is also near the internal carotid artery.

The *maxillary division* supplies the palate, upper jaw, upper teeth, cheek and maxillary sinuses. It enters the skull through the foramen rotundum.

The *mandibular division* supplies the lower jaw, lower teeth and anterior two thirds of the tongue. It has a motor branch which

Figure 7 Sensory innervation of the head and face.
The distribution of the trigeminal nerve and its branches are shown

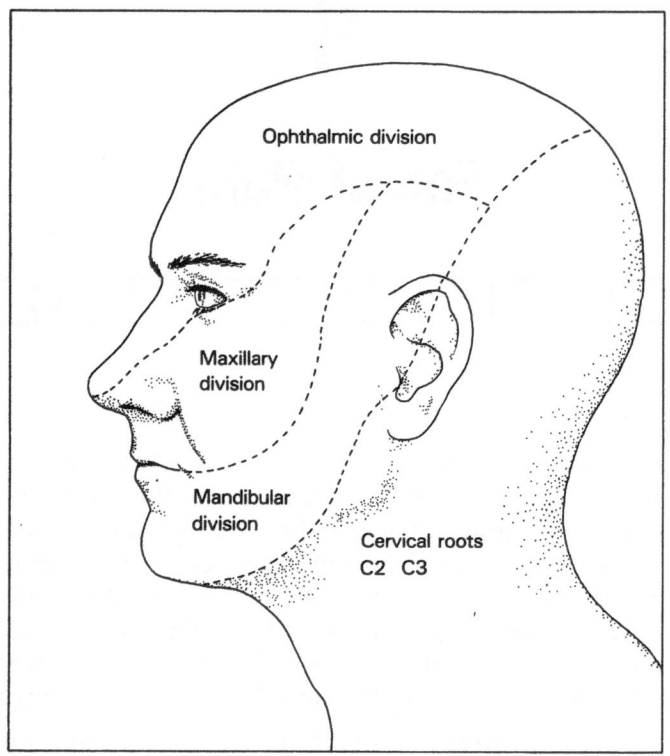

supplies the temporalis and masseter muscles. It enters the skull through the foramen ovale.

ACUTE FACIAL PAIN

Dental disease

This is the most common cause of acute facial pain. It may arise as:

(1) Hypersensitivity – triggered by hot, cold and sweetness.

(2) Pulpitic – often hard to localise, particularly if the patient has many fillings.

(3) Inflammatory – usually throbbing severe pain associated with local tenderness. This may lead to abscess formation with further soft tissue swelling and a purulent discharge[18].

Dental referral is necessary although analgesics and antibiotics may be prescribed. Infections are often streptococcal in origin with sometimes added anaerobes so penicillin, amoxycillin (Amoxil) and metronidazole (Flagyl) may be useful.

Sinus infection (page 33)

This may be a pan-sinusitis or local sinus disease. Maxillary sinusitis may mimic dental pain, and conversely an apical dental abscess may provoke maxillary sinusitis. Commonly there is throbbing facial pain, the site determined by the sinus involved. This may be worsened by movement or bending. Often there is accompanying nasal obstruction and a purulent discharge, although the last may be absent if the ostium of the antrum is blocked. There may be local tenderness. X-rays will confirm the diagnosis.

Treatment includes antibiotics – commonly penicillin or amoxycillin (Amoxil). Erythromycin may be used if there is a history of penicillin allergy. Analgesics and nasal decongestants may also be helpful. The last include menthol inhalations and ½% ephedrine nasal drops. Failure to respond requires hospital referral.

Ocular inflammation (page 33)

This is often associated with a painful red eye with a fall in visual acuity. Ophthalmological referral is necessary if acute glaucoma or uveitis are suspected.

Herpes zoster ophthalmicus

This is the commonest site for shingles. It presents acutely with pain in the forehead and eye. Within three to four days a herpetic skin eruption appears. The eyelids may become very swollen and the eye painful and inflamed.

Urgent referral to an ophthalmologist is necessary as patients may develop corneal damage from the sensory loss, iritis with secondary glaucoma, involvement of the optic nerve and even extraocular muscle palsies.

Trauma

This is usually self-evident from the history, soft tissue bruising and swelling. Good quality X-rays of the facial bones may be necessary. Any facial fractures may require referral to a maxillo-facial specialist.

Giant cell arteritis (page 28)

This may involve the facial artery with pain in the face aggravated by chewing.

RECURRENT FACIAL PAIN

These pains are common, particularly migraine and its variants, and trigeminal neuralgia.

Migraine

Classical migraine has already been described (page 21) but in some patients facial pain associated with headache is prominent. This is usually unilateral and may spread into the neck.

Migrainous neuralgia (cluster headache)

Here recurrent episodes of intense distressing pain occur, centred in or around the orbit, lasting 30–60 minutes. The pain is associated with oculosympathetic disturbance so there may be ipsilateral ptosis, miosis, conjunctival suffusion, epiphora and nasal stuffiness. The patient, usually a middle aged man, complains of recurring episodes (a cluster) of pain awaking him from sleep on successive nights over a period of 3 to 4 weeks. The cluster then may abate spontaneously. A few patients have several episodes of pain within 24 hours. Alcohol may precipitate an attack. Often such patients give no history of typical migraine.

Treatment

A Cafergot suppository (ergotamine 2 mg and caffeine 100 mg) inserted at bed-time for five successive nights will usually control an attack. The dose is omitted on the sixth night. If the pain returns, treatment is continued for another five nights. Oral ergot preparations may be disappointing and injections have now been discontinued.

Oral treatment helps some patients. It is only necessary for the duration of the cluster. Such treatment includes:

(1) Pizotifen (Sanomigran) 0.5 mg b.d. increasing to 3 mg/day.

(2) Methysergide (Deseril) 1 mg b.d. increasing to 2 mg t.i.d. This should not be used continuously for more than 16 weeks because of the small risks of retroperitoneal fibrosis.

(3) Lithium (Camcolit, Priadel) 250 mg b.d. to start. Usually only a low dose is necessary and blood levels should not exceed 1.2 mmol/l although most patients respond at levels of 0.6 mmol/l. Lithium should not be used in patients with renal insufficiency or cardiovascular disease, and care should be taken if patients are receiving diuretics.

Migrainous variants

These include *'Lower half headache'*, sphenopalatine and vidian neuralgia. Here attacks of facial pain arise in the cheek, palate and angle of the nose. The pain may spread into the whole face, or even radiate behind the ear or into the neck and shoulder on one side. The pain may last hours or a day and may be associated with nausea and photophobia. In some attacks patients feel the cheek is swollen and tender.

Patients often respond to pizotifen, methysergide or other antimigrainous preparations (page 24).

Chronic paroxysmal hemicrania

This is uncommon but may present as brief attacks of severe pain usually in the temple or orbit on one side lasting 20–30 minutes[14]. These may be repeated several times daily. Another variant consists of multiple jabs of pain differing in severity and location.

Such patients may respond to indomethacin (Indocid) 25 mg t.i.d. or q.i.d. This sometimes may cause indigestion or even provoke headache.

Benign coital cephalgia

Recurring throbbing headache may occur with facial pain sometimes provoked by exertion or coitus. Acute coital headache may arise from a sub-arachnoid haemorrhage particularly in the hypertensive. More often it is a benign entity causing considerable distress[15].

Exertional headache may respond to indomethacin (75 mg/day) and benign coital cephalgia may be helped by propranolol (Inderal) 120–180 mg/day.

Trigeminal neuralgia *(Tic Douloureux)*

Symptoms

The diagnosis rests on the description of the pain. This is very severe, stabbing with repeated jabs, usually lasting seconds only. It is localised in the territory of the maxillary and mandibular divisions on one side. It is commonly triggered by touch, movement, washing, shaving, eating or temperature. If the stabs are very frequent patients become fearful of any activity which may provoke pain, leading the life of an invalid. Such episodes may last weeks or months and then be followed by long periods of freedom. During and between episodes there are no abnormal signs. Most patients are elderly, and women are more often affected. In some patients between the jabs of pain, there may be a background of more constant facial discomfort. The cause is usually unknown.

In some patients trigeminal neuralgia may be *symptomatic*. In younger patients it may be a symptom of multiple sclerosis. Even more rarely it may be provoked by a cerebellopontine angle tumour or basilar aneurysm. In such instances, however, there is often trigeminal sensory loss and other signs of cranial nerve involvement or of cerebellar upset.

Glossopharyngeal neuralgia

Similar acute stabbing neuralgic pains may also arise in the territory of the glossopharyngeal nerve. The pain is felt on one side of the throat or in the ear and may be triggered by swallowing.

Treatment

Two thirds of patients with trigeminal neuralgia will respond to carbamezepine (Tegretol). In the elderly start with a low dose – 100 mg b.d. and gradually increase this until the pain is controlled. Often a dose of 200 mg q.i.d. is necessary but occasional patients will require higher doses – up to 1600 mg daily. Once the pain has been controlled, the dose can be reduced. High doses of carbamazepine may cause unsteadiness and double vision. Very rarely marrow depression has occurred.

Other drugs may be tried: phenytoin (Epanutin) – 100 mg t.i.d. or clonazepam (Rivotril) 2 – 6 mg daily. Either of these in high dose may cause unsteadiness and drowsiness.

Surgical treatment

In patients who fail to respond to medical treatment, referral to a neurosurgeon or pain clinic may be necessary. In younger patients partial nerve root section or micro-decompression of the exposed trigeminal nerve may give relief although these measures require a craniotomy. In older patients chemical injection or thermocoagulation of the ganglion or its main branches may afford relief, but usually at the price of persisting facial sensory loss. After surgery or injection a small number of patients complain bitterly of the perisistent sensory upset – anaesthesia dolorosa.

CHRONIC FACIAL PAIN

This may arise from a number of uncommon but serious causes. Often there is pain in association with:

(1) An ophthalmoplegia, failing vision or proptosis. This suggests an orbital lesion – a tumour, granuloma or aneurysm (page 101).

(2) Sensory loss commonly in the maxillary division. This may be associated with a swelling in the throat, nasal passage obstruction and sometimes cranial nerve involvement. These suggest a nasopharyngeal carcinoma or lymphoma.

(3) Lower cranial nerve involvement (and sometimes double vision). This may arise from a tumour eroding the skull base. Tumours include a chordoma, metastasis, meningioma and neuroma as well as those in (2) above.

Such patients require hospital referral. Plain X-rays of the skull, orbits and basal views may show bone erosion. An ESR may be helpful, particularly if a granuloma is suspected.

Post-herpetic neuralgia

Following an attack of zoster ophthalmicus about 15% of patients may develop chronic distressing pain at the site of the previous infection. This may have left residual scarring of the skin with some disturbance of sensation. The pain is persistent, fluctuating in severity and of variable pattern. It responds poorly to simple analgesics. Affected patients are often elderly and lonely. Many become depressed. They try to avoid contact with the affected area of the face.

Treatment

This involves the regular use of simple analgesics together with an anti-depressant given as a single dose at bed-time, e.g. trimipramine (Surmontil) 25–75 mg nocte. Another combination which may prove helpful is amitriptyline (Tryptizol) 25 mg t.i.d. with fluphenazine (Moditen) 1 mg t.i.d. In the very elderly the doses may need to be reduced.

Simple physical measures should also be tried; advising patients to touch, rub and even vibrate the skin of the affected area. Treatment is often disappointing and patients may need referral to a pain clinic.

Temporo-mandibular joint dysfunction *(Costen's syndrome)*

This produces pain usually in front of the ear which may spread to the temple, face and neck. The pain is often aggravated by chewing and may be associated with an audible clicking of the jaw joint. Malocclusion of the bite is a feature so there are complaints of difficulty with jaw movements, and sometimes of 'locking'. Younger women are most often affected.

Referral to a *dental specialist* is necessary and treatment is often a combination of a muscle relaxant as diazepam (Valium) and the use of a night bite appliance[13].

ATYPICAL FACIAL PAIN

Most often this is seen in middle aged women who bitterly complain of persistent facial pain described in superlatives, arising deep in the cheek. The site is variable and the pain may fluctuate in intensity. It seems to be little affected by simple analgesics. There are no abnormal signs but many patients appear depressed.

Many such patients are referred to dentists, ophthalmologists, ENT surgeons, and eventually neurologists. The diagnosis is one of exclusion.

Treatment is disappointing. Explanation and reassurance together with an anti-depressant may help some patients.

BELL'S PALSY

Symptoms and signs

This is usually a painless lower motor neurone facial paralysis of one side of the face of acute onset. This may come on over 24–28 hours and may be partial or complete. In complete lesions the eye cannot be closed and there is a danger of corneal exposure damage. The palpebral fissure on the affected side appears wider and there is loss or paucity of blinking. Tears may spill over the lower lid. The side of the mouth is crooked, the cheek flaccid and food may accumulate in the cheek.

There may be pain or discomfort behind the ear at the onset. If the cause is an ear infection or attack of herpes zoster then there may be pain in the ear.

If the part of the facial nerve distal to the chorda tympani is involved then there may be loss of taste in the anterior two thirds of the tongue on the affected side. Occasionally patients may complain of increased loudness of sounds in the affected ear.

Prognosis

The palsy commonly arises as an acute inflammation of the facial nerve causing local demyelination with a conduction block. In some 15% of patients the damage is more severe and axonal degeneration of the nerve may follow. If this has occurred repair must then be by regeneration which is slow, often incomplete and may lead to aberrant re-innervation with jaw-winking (mouth movement causes eye closure). If demyelination has occurred, recovery usually follows over a period of some weeks. If some recovery has appeared by three weeks from the onset, it is likely there will be good recovery.

Causes

There is an increased incidence in hypertension, diabetes and multiple sclerosis. Rarely the palsy may be bilateral and this may occur in acute polyneuritis, sarcoidosis or neoplastic infiltration. Geniculate zoster infections may be associated with vesicles in the external auditory meatus, acute deafness and often vertigo as well as the facial palsy.

Treatment

The role of steroids is controversial. It has been suggested that their use early in the disease may reduce swelling of the facial nerve and so prevent axonal degeneration. In patients seen within seven days of onset, prednisolone 40–60 mg daily given for five days may be used and the dose then rapidly reduced.

EMG studies performed five days or more after the onset, may be valuable in predicting patients where axonal degeneration has occurred, i.e. those who are likely to make a slow and incomplete recovery.

6

Visual Disturbances

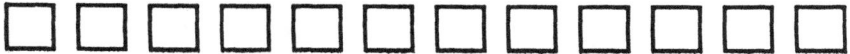

All patients with complaints of visual upset should have their acuity for distance (Snellen) and close work (reading) measured (page 8). Refractive errors are the commonest cause of a low acuity and can easily be checked using a pinhole (page 9).

Colour vision Although some patients are colour blind (usually red–green), inability to read Ishihara or similar test type cards may indicate an acquired fault in the optic nerve or retina.

Macular lesions Central (macular) visual faults cause a significant drop in acuity. Patients may be aware of these as positive scotomata and they may be demonstrated by the use of Amsler charts. The chart consists of a grid pattern on a card which when held about 30 cms from the patient, will test the central twenty degrees of the field. Most local macular and retinal lesions are visible with the ophthalmoscope (although the pupil may need to be dilated for a good view of the macula).

ACUTE VISUAL FAILURE

Eye causes

Ophthalmic causes are often *vascular* as in *retinal artery* or *vein occlusions*, or *vitreous haemorrhage*[16]. These cause painless visual loss progressing over minutes or hours. Patients are often elderly and may show signs of vascular disease, e.g. hypertension. Diabetes and giant cell arteritis are other conditions which need exclusion. *Retinal detachment* may also cause painless acute visual loss with the appearance of a 'cloud or shadow' in the field of vision. Many patients complain of floaters, light flashes or spots in their eyes, at the onset. Patients show a drop in acuity which is marked if the macula is involved, field loss (commonly noticed by the patient) and retinal changes. All such patients require urgent referral to an ophthalmologist.

Acute optic neuritis (retro-bulbar neuritis)

This is caused by inflammation of the optic nerve (demyelination). Younger patients are commonly affected (aged 18–50) who complain of visual blurring or loss, progressing over hours or days. Often there is tenderness of the globe and pain on eye movement. Some patients are aware that the visual loss is worse in bright light, after exercise or a hot bath. Rarely both eyes may be affected together or sequentially.

Causes In more than half such patients with prolonged follow-up there may be other episodes of neurological disturbance to suggest a diagnosis of multiple sclerosis (MS). Some patients have an isolated episode, others repeated attacks. Patients with established MS commonly have attacks of optic neuritis. Very rarely an optic neuritis may occur in glandular fever, sarcoidosis, syphilis, and zoster ophthalmicus.

Signs In optic neuritis patients show a depressed acuity (from 6/9 to light perception) with usually a central field loss. There is an afferent pupillary defect (page 10) and impaired colour vision. Commonly the retina and optic nerve appear normal but in a small number the nerve head, the papilla, is inflamed and swollen – papillitis (similar in appearance to papilloedema but there is a marked fall in acuity).

In approximately 90% of patients there is spontaneous recovery with vision returning to near normal (at least 6/9) commonly within three to six weeks. After the episode an afferent pupillary defect and impaired colour vision persist. Sometimes pallor of the optic disc appears suggesting optic atrophy. Measurement of VEP's will show significant prolongation of latency in an affected optic nerve and this delay persists after the attack.

Treatment In many instances a course of steroids (ACTH injections, tablets or even retro-orbital injection) have been used. These do not alter the outcome in terms of the degree of recovery but may bring that recovery earlier.

Ischaemic papillitis

This may arise in older patients who often have signs of vascular disease. It may also occur in giant cell arteritis. Usually there is an acute vascular occlusion of the ciliary and/or central retinal arteries supplying the optic nerve, which produces acute visual loss, either total or partial. In the latter there is often an altitudinal field defect. The visual loss is painless. The optic disc appears swollen and pale with thin attenuated vessels. An ESR should be set up immediately and urgent referral to hospital is necessary because there may be an arteritis. In many patients, however, the visual loss persists.

TRANSIENT VISUAL UPSETS

Brief episodes of visual upset may occur in migraine: these often last 15–45 minutes and are followed by severe headache. Momentary obscurations of vision may occur with very high intracranial pressure, usually triggered by bending, coughing or exercise.

Amaurosis fugax describes episodes of monocular visual loss often lasting 1–2 minutes which patients liken to a 'shutter or curtain' coming down over their field of vision. Sometimes retinal emboli may be visible during an episode.

Ocular causes

Acute glaucoma may produce acute painful loss of vision progressing over a few hours. Haloes may be seen around objects at first. The pain is intense and may be accompanied by vomiting. The eye is red, the acuity depressed and the pupil enlarged. Urgent referral to an eye clinic is necessary. *Uveitis* may also cause visual blurring with local eye discomfort and a red eye.

COMPRESSION OF THE OPTIC NERVE

This is often painless and patients may present with progressive visual loss. Initially there may be a central scotoma which then spreads peripherally, some patients seem very slow to recognise that vision is failing in one eye. Depending on the site of compression other structures will be involved with the appearance of other symptoms and signs.

At the apex of the orbit (Figure 8), masses may arise. These include neuromas, cavernous angiomas, metastases, lymphomas and granulómas. At this site a mass will cause proptosis and often limitation of the full range of eye movements with the complaint of diplopia.

The most common site of compression is behind the orbit often from a meningioma (from the anterior clinoid process or lesser wing of sphenoid). There may also be compression within the cavernous sinus (Figure 8). At this site the optic nerve runs close to the 3,4 and 6 cranial nerves, and the first division of the trigeminal nerve so that there may be complaints of double vision, ptosis and even facial numbness.

Chiasmal compression Compression at this site most often arises from below from an enlarging pituitary tumour. Classically the visual loss is bitemporal in approximately 60% and unilateral blindness with a contralateral temporal field cut in approximately 15% (Figure 9). The visual loss in one eye may not be noticed by the patient until vision in the second eye is failing.

Figure 8 Diagram of the left orbit from above to show the orbital and retro-orbital structures with cranial nerves 3, 4, 5 and 6 and the carotid artery

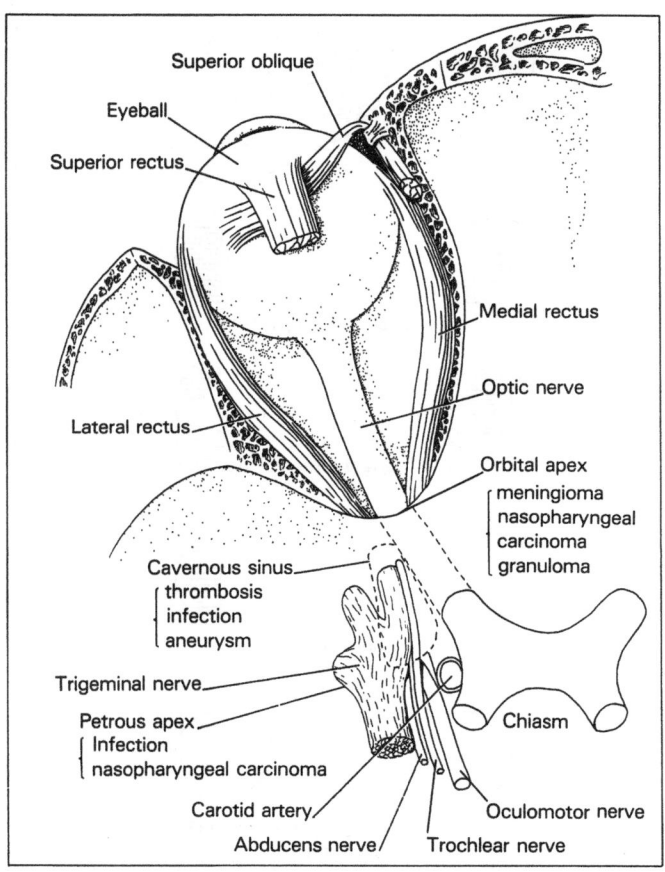

Pituitary lesions may produce signs and symptoms of endocrine failure or overactivity. Hypopituitarism is more common with amenorrhoea, impotence and infertility often as first symptoms. More florid signs include a curious waxy pallor, smooth skin with loss of body hair and even florid myxoedema. Hypersecreting pituitary tumours may cause acromegaly, Cushing's syndrome or even prolactin excess – these are rare.

Figure 9 Field defects from chiasmal compression

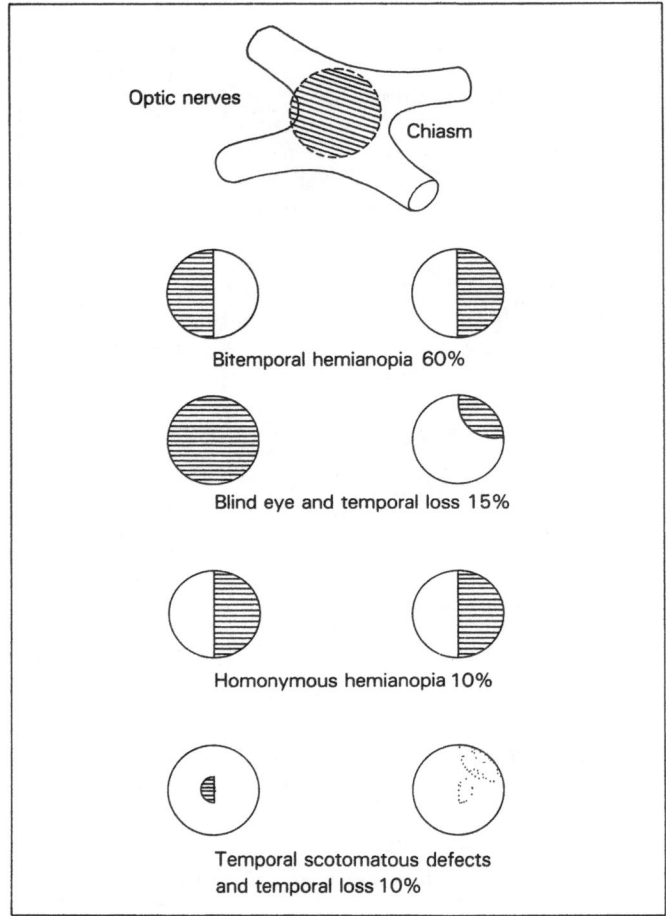

RETRO-CHIASMAL VISUAL PATHWAY DAMAGE

This includes damage to the optic tract and radiation which will produce a *homonymous hemianopia* or *quadrantanopia* (Figure 4) in the contralateral field. Congruous field defects suggest more posteriorly placed damage. A hemianopia may pass unnoticed by a patient, particularly if they are confused, a feature which may occur after a stroke or with a cerebral tumour, the two commonest causes of hemianopia. Sometimes there are complaints of difficulty reading as they miss one side of the page; other patients may have accidents driving or walk into the side of a doorframe in their blind half field.

Confrontation techniques (Figure 3) will detect most hemianopic defects. The acuity in the good half of the field is often normal but patients sometimes miss one side of the Snellen chart.

Cortical blindness results from bilateral occipital cortex damage, usually from bilateral posterior cerebral artery lesions, often thrombotic. Patients appear confused, may seem unaware of their visual defect and have normal pupillary reactions. Many show a sector of preserved vision in their fields which they may use. Some mistakenly are labelled as 'functional'.

Patients with such field defects require hospital referral.

CHRONIC VISUAL LOSS

Ocular causes

Slow visual loss usually arises from ophthalmic causes[16], particularly *glaucoma*, and in the elderly *cataract* and *macular degeneration*. *Diabetes* may also damage the retina causing progressive visual loss, and this is the commonest cause of blindness in patients aged 30–65. In all these patients, the acuity, fields, lens changes and retinal appearances often give the diagnosis but such patients need ophthalmic referral.

Toxic damage may occur to the optic nerves. The causes include tobacco, alcohol, poisons (e.g. methyl alcohol) and drugs (e.g. ethambutol (Myambutol), quinine, chloramphenicol (Chloromycetin), and chloroquine (Avloclor, Nivaquine)). Vitamin B12 deficiency may also cause optic atrophy.

Rare *inherited forms* of optic atrophy also occur. Here there is usually a family history. The most common is Leber's; this predominantly affects males.

In all patients with unexplained optic atrophy it is worth taking a blood sample for B12 estimation and WR (or equivalent). Skull X-rays may show an enlarged pituitary fossa or intracranial calcification.

DOUBLE VISION

Patients may show evidence of an obvious squint with one eye turned in (convergent) or one eye turned out (divergent). This may occur if there is a longstanding amblyopic eye; some 5% of the British population have an amblyopic eye. The onset of diplopia suggests a break-down of the yoked gaze of the two eyes in parallel. The rules for the assessment of diplopia – finding the direction of maximal separation of images and applying the cover test – have already been described (page 13). It is often possible by observation of volitional (willed) eye movements and then pursuit (following) movements to detect the fault. Longstanding defects may be accompanied by a head tilt or turning. Cover testing of each eye in turn will show a latent or true squint. Apley[17] suggests that in *young children* with a squint three tests should be made: (1) to measure the acuity in both eyes, (2) to assess the intelligence and (3) to examine the nervous system. In about one quarter of children with a squint there are signs of cerebral dysfunction.

OCULAR MOTOR PALSIES

These involve damage to the sixth, third and fourth cranial nerves, in that order of frequency. A sixth nerve palsy causes failure of abduction of the affected eye due to paralysis of the lateral rectus muscle (Figure 10). A complete oculomotor palsy causes ptosis with an enlarged pupil in an eye that has lost all movements apart from abduction (Figure 11). The movements are described in Table 6. The most common causes in the young are trauma, MS, tumours and aneurysms. In the old, vascular disease (diabetes), aneurysms, tumours (include nasopharyngeal carcinoma) and

Figure 10 Right abducens palsy

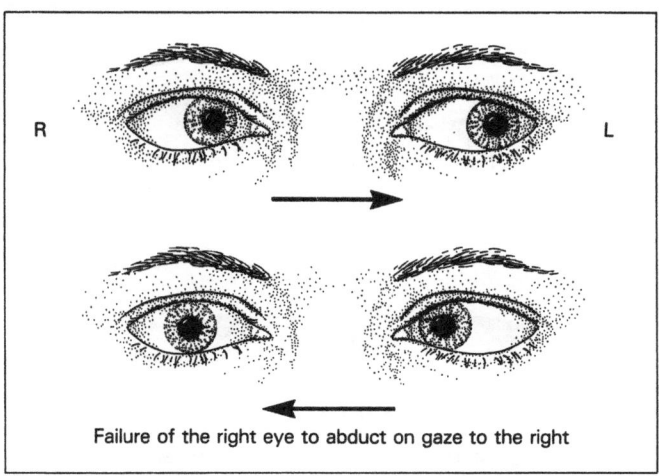

R L

Failure of the right eye to abduct on gaze to the right

trauma may be responsible. Pain is likely to occur with vascular lesions (arteritic, diabetic, occlusive and aneurysmal) and with granulomas causing nerve damage.

DYSTHYROID EYE DISEASE

One of the common causes of double vision in the middle aged is from thyroid upset. This most often presents with vertical diplopia from restriction of upgaze (due to tethering of the inferior rectus) and less commonly from tethering of the medial rectus simulating an abducens palsy. The eye often appears proptosed with lid lag and some conjunctival congestion (Figure 12). Any suspicion merits a *blood sample* for *thyroid function tests*.

MYASTHENIA GRAVIS

This may present with variable diplopia which alternates affecting different eye muscles on separate occasions. It is often worse in the

Figure 11 Right oculomotor palsy

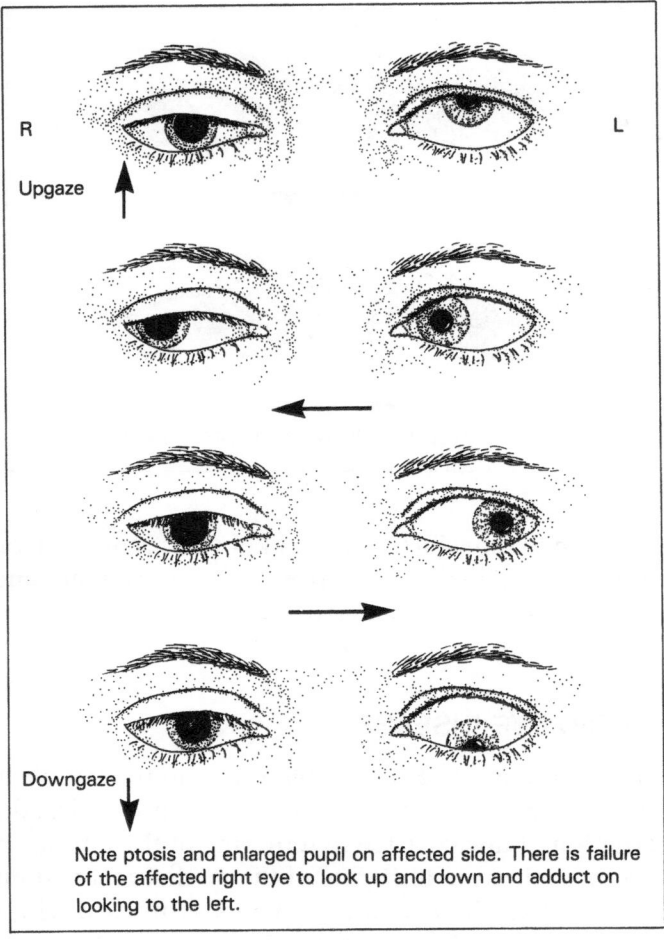

R

Upgaze

L

Downgaze

Note ptosis and enlarged pupil on affected side. There is failure of the affected right eye to look up and down and adduct on looking to the left.

evenings and may be associated with variable ptosis and weakness of eyelid closure. Many patients also have symptoms of bulbar and facial muscle weakness and of a proximal myopathy (page 143).

An edrophonium (Tensilon) test will confirm the diagnosis. Edrophonium is a short acting anti-cholinesterase. 2 mg are given intravenously and the effect checked. If there is no upset, then the

Figure 12 Dysthyroid eye disease

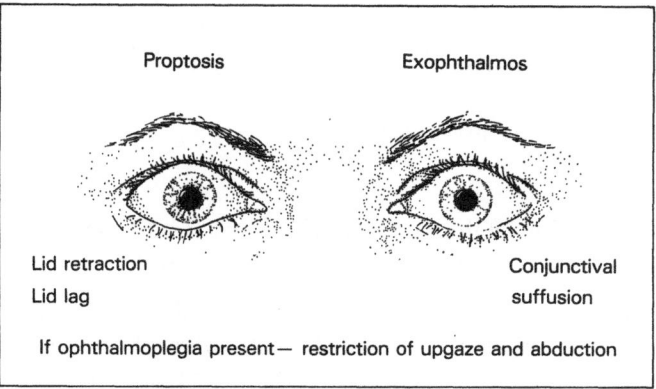

remaining 8 mg are given (1 ampoule holds 10 mg). A positive response appears within 1 – 2 minutes with loss of ptosis and return of the full range of eye movements. The injection may produce transient muscle flickering, nausea and tears.

Such patients will require referral to a neurologist.

Children with double vision

If there is no history of trauma a careful examination should always be made, checking there are no signs of raised intracranial pressure, cerebellar upset or enlargement of the expected skull circumference. Posterior fossa tumours may present with diplopia. Some children may show a head tilt. Such children require specialist referral.

CONJUGATE GAZE PROBLEMS

Within the brain stem lie the nuclei of the third, fourth and sixth cranial nerves. These are connected by a number of pathways producing yoked movements of the two eyes. They are under the

97

influence of a number of other centres – posterior frontal, occipital, basal ganglia and pons (oculo-vestibular). Destructive or irritative lesions in these central pathways cause derangements of conjugate eye movements and gaze palsies. A *gaze palsy* is the inability to move the eyes, either by volitional or following movements, past the mid-line in any given direction.

MEDIAL LONGITUDINAL FASCICULUS (MLF) AND INTERNUCLEAR OPHTHALMOPLEGIA (INO)

The MLF connects the pontine centres (sixth nerve) with the oculomotor nuclei at the level of the colliculi and is responsible for the yoked horizontal movements of the eyes (medial rectus on one side with the lateral rectus on the other). Damage to the MLF, as most often occurs with MS or strokes, produces an INO with failure of adduction of the eye on the affected side and coarse ataxic nystagmus in the abducting eye (away from the affected side Figure 13). The INO may be bilateral and then is most often due to MS.

Figure 13 Right internuclear ophthalmoplegia

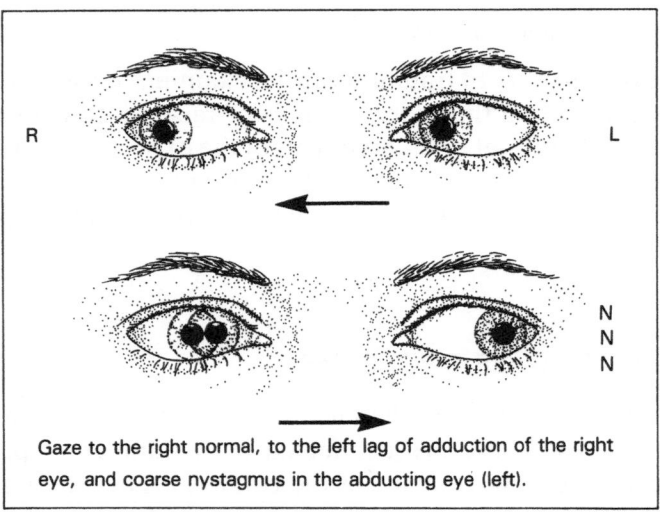

Gaze to the right normal, to the left lag of adduction of the right eye, and coarse nystagmus in the abducting eye (left).

Figures 14(a),(b),(c) Supranuclear gaze palsies

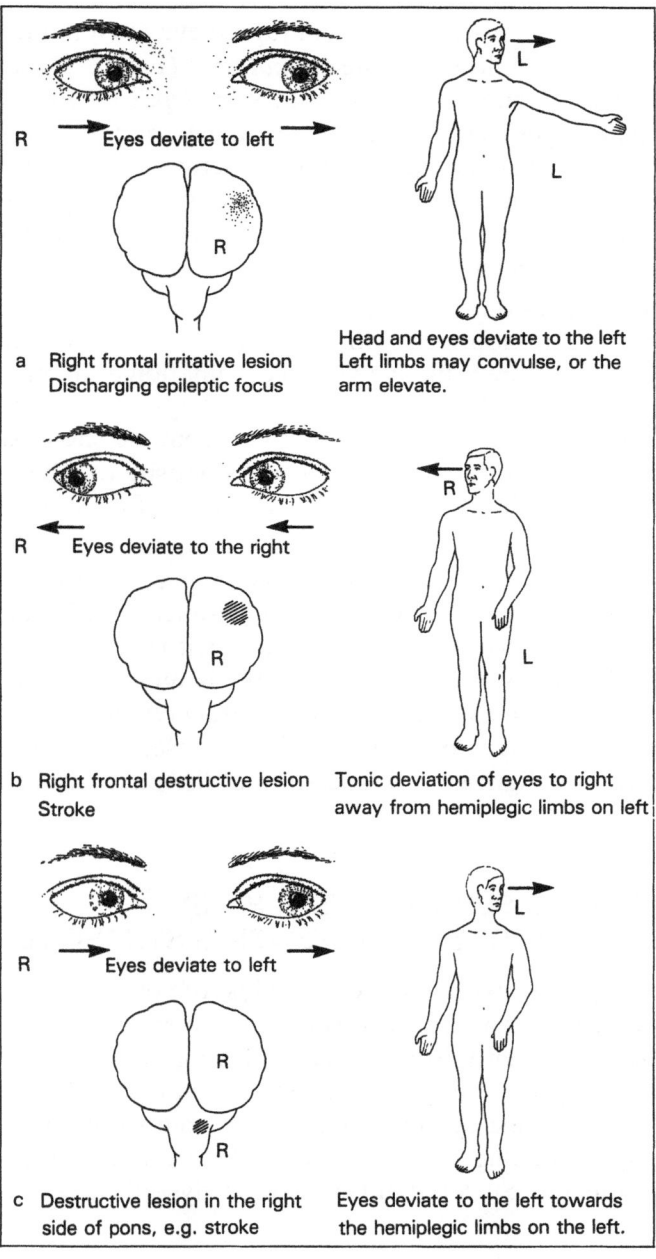

R → Eyes deviate to left →

R

Head and eyes deviate to the left
Left limbs may convulse, or the
arm elevate.

a   Right frontal irritative lesion
Discharging epileptic focus

R ← Eyes deviate to the right ←

R

Tonic deviation of eyes to right
away from hemiplegic limbs on left

b   Right frontal destructive lesion
Stroke

R → Eyes deviate to left →

R

R

Eyes deviate to the left towards
the hemiplegic limbs on the left.

c   Destructive lesion in the right
side of pons, e.g. stroke

SUPRANUCLEAR LESIONS

Supranuclear lesions disturbing conjugate eye movements do not usually produce diplopia. In the *frontal* area (Figure 21) an irritative lesion at this site, as may occur in an *epileptic seizure*, will turn the head and eyes to the opposite side, away from the discharging focus (Figure 14a). Conversely a destructive lesion at the same site, as may occur with a *stroke*, will allow deviation of the head and eyes towards the side of the frontal lobe damage, that is away from the hemiplegic limbs (Figure 14b).

Destructive lesions in the *pons*, usually from strokes, but occasionally from tumours or MS, are more often associated with diplopia. Here there is likely to be a combination of damage to the ocular motor and other cranial nerves with nystagmus. There may be conjugate deviation of the eyes away from the site of damage, towards the side of the hemiplegia (the opposite to a hemisphere lesion) (Figure 14c). Such patients appear ill often showing cerebellar as well as pyramidal tract signs.

Conjugate *vertical* eye movements may also show irritative upsets, as in oculogyric crisis – seen in post-encephalitic Parkinsonism, and the effects of destructive lesions, with paralysis of upward gaze (Parinaud's syndrome). The latter is most often seen with tumours (pinealomas) but also with hydrocephalus, MS and even vascular lesions. Such patients often show absence of convergence of the eyes and light-near dissociation of the pupillary responses.

PROGRESSIVE SUPRANUCLEAR PALSY (STEELE–RICHARDSON–OLSZEWSKI'S SYNDROME)

This is a degenerative disease causing loss of neurones in the basal ganglia and mid-brain. Because such patients show extrapyramidal signs they are often misdiagnosed as having Parkinson's disease. Loss of conjugate vertical eye movements, particularly downgaze, is often the earliest symptom leading to complaints of difficulty with vision in reading. Later upgaze and horizontal eye movements are also affected. Such patients may show dysarthria, axial rigidity (particularly the face and neck), dementia and pyramidal signs. The condition progresses with a steady physical deterioration and shows a very poor response to anti-Parkinsonian drugs.

OCULAR MYOPATHIES

These are rare causes of restricted eye movements with an insidious onset, slow progression and often no complaints of diplopia. There may also be ptosis. In many there is a positive family history and a dominant inheritance. Very rarely an 'ophthalmoplegia plus' may arise with an external ophthalmoplegia and evidence of more widespread damage as heart block, retinitis pigmentosa and even pathological changes in skeletal muscle. Hospital referral will be necessary.

PROPTOSIS WITH OPHTHALMOPLEGIA
(ALL WITH ABNORMAL EYE MOVEMENTS)

(1) *Trauma* Obvious 'black eye', may be associated orbit fracture if diplopia is present.

(2) *Infective* Facial sepsis or septicaemia may cause an acute orbital cellulitis or cavernous sinus thrombosis. Marked local inflammatory swelling with chemosis. May lead to irreversible visual loss. Patients need urgent admission.

(3) *Tumour* A mass within the orbit may displace the globe and restrict eye movements. Causes include a metastasis, spread from a naso-pharyngeal carcinoma, lymphoma, cavernous angioma, neuroma, neuroblastoma (children), meningioma or lachrymal gland tumour.

(4) *Granuloma* This may arise with a 'painful ophthalmoplegia' (Tolosa Hunt syndrome) associated with systemic upset and a high ESR. This is very steroid responsive. Other causes include sarcoidosis and Wegener's granuloma.

(5) *Carotico-cavernous fistula* This may follow trauma or even appear spontaneously. It produces a pulsating proptosis with very congested eye. A bruit is audible.

(6) *Dysthyroid eye disease* (page 95).

All these conditions require specialist referral.

7

Failing Memory

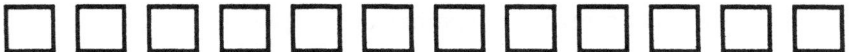

DEFINITION

This is the loss of ability to remember recent and/or distant events. There is usually an inability to learn new material. Failing memory may be associated with a decline in alertness, reasoning and problem-solving skills. There may also be loss of perception, impaired comprehension and speech, and difficulties in reading and writing. As this progresses there is a loss of all skills, a global dementia. Dementia usually arises from diffuse neuronal disturbance leading to widespread changes in personality and behaviour, as well as memory impairment. As the condition progresses there is physical deterioration with wandering, neglect of personal appearance and often incontinence.

FOCAL LESIONS

It is important to realise that focal cerebral lesions, as a tumour or stroke, may present with changes in higher cerebral function. Furthermore some patients with cerebral tumours may show a focal onset but as the lesion increases in size, more widespread disturbance may occur with increasing drowsiness and confusion.

Multiple cerebral metastases may present with widespread changes in higher mental functions.

Focal cerebral deficits causing problems include:

Dominant hemisphere lesions with speech disturbance

A severe dysphasia with problems in comprehension and expression may be mistaken for dementia. There are often problems in spelling, writing, reading and calculating. Two main sites of dominant hemisphere damage (usually the left) are found causing rather different patterns of dysphasia.

Dysphasia

(1) *Broca's* – non-fluent or expressive. Speech here is slow, hesitant with poor articulation. The content is telegrammatic and patients may show difficulty in saying "No, ifs, ands or buts". Comprehension is usually spared.

(2) *Wernicke's* – fluent or receptive. Speech may be rapid and seems fluent although in content there may be errors, omitted words and circumlocutions. Often there is some loss of understanding.

In Broca's dysphasia the site is in the posterior part of the frontal lobe by the inferior frontal gyrus (Figure 15). In Wernicke's dysphasia the site is in the temporal lobe around the angular gyrus[18].

Parietal and parieto-occipital lobe lesions

These may cause visual and sensory disturbances in the contralateral side of the body and limbs. These include sensory inattention (including the visual field), neglect and even denial that the affected part belongs to the patient. These are most common in right parietal lesions. Bilateral and sometimes right parieto-occipital lesions may also cause problems in finding the way, in

Figure 15 Lateral surface of the cerebral hemisphere to show speech areas

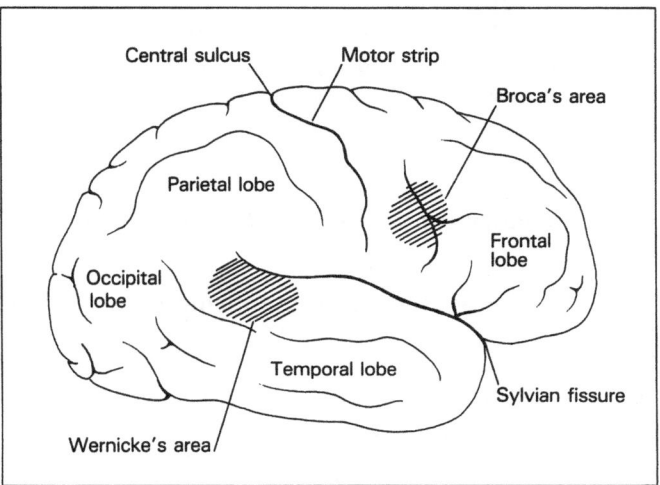

·dressing, drawing and constructing figures and even recognition of faces. Many posteriorly placed lesions produce a contralateral hemianopia.

Frontal lobe lesions

These are likely to cause changes in personality and behaviour often much more apparent to relatives than the patient. Usually there is also a decline in intellectual skills and problems in making decisions, in planning and concentrating. Many patients show perseveration in thought and speech. Smell may be lost with some frontal tumours.

BRAIN FAILURE

In recent years the term brain failure has become fashionable, replacing the word dementia. Advanced brain failure has been defined as the end stage of a syndrome characterised by impaired social functioning due to the inability to learn because of a decline of intellect. This is judged to be present when, because of impaired memory, the patient is unable to cope with independent social living despite having the normal physical ability to do so[29]. It is a functional definition and is classified into mild, moderate and severe[10].

Mild

(1) Loss of memory for recent trivial information.

(2) Occasional loss of orientation.

(3) Capable of living alone and organising their own affairs.

Moderate

(1) Loss of memory for recent trivial information.

(2) Occasional loss of orientation.

(3) Difficulty in concentration.

(4) Fluctuating disorientation.

(5) Tendency to become confused and restless.

(6) Possible incontinence.

(7) Incapable of living alone.

(8) Require almost constant supervision.

Severe

(1) Incapable of coherent or sustained speech, or of indicating or responding to commands.

(2) Totally dependent. Nearly always require hospitalisation.

What problems arise?

(1) Recognition of the loss by the patient, those about the patient – friends, relatives and the doctor.

(2) Difficulties of assessment.
(a) Knowledge of premorbid personality, intelligence and interests.
(b) The available tests are crude.

(c) Associated conditions which may mask the condition – blindness, deafness, social isolation, depression and delusions.

(d) Associated illnesses causing the loss – hypothyroidism, vitamin B12 deficiency, etc.

(3) What is the exact diagnosis? Is it remediable? How far to investigate?

(4) Management – this will depend on the patient's willingness to accept that there is a problem and take appropriate measures. The patient will have to be assessed in relation to his daily living, mobility and medical care. Support for the patient may need to be organised. The prognosis may need to be discussed with the patient and their reactions explored.

(5) The rising incidence with age is placing an increasing burden on health care resources.

Aetiology

Some 15% of the causes are potentially reversible; some 85% are not because they are due to nerve cell loss either by degeneration or other damage.

Commonest by far	senile dementia and Alzheimer's disease
Common	arteriosclerosis – multiple infarcts
	alcohol
	multiple sclerosis
	drugs
	toxic confusional states
Uncommon but important	vitamin deficiencies – B12, B1 (Wernicke's encephalopathy), folate deficiency
	hypothyroidism
	Huntington's chorea (page 166)
	frontal lobe tumours

107

trauma – brain damage, subdural haematoma, punch-drunk boxers or steeple-chase jockeys

normal pressure hydrocephalus (page 110)

syphilis

uraemia

Rare   Jakob–Creutzfeldt's disease (slow virus infection)

cerebral lipidosis (children).

Senile dementia and Alzheimer's disease

This has a prevalence of 6% at 65 years and 20% at 80 years. There is no sex difference; the apparent predominance of females is due to the fact that there are less old men alive. Isolation, malnutrition and poor social conditions may occur as a result of the illness but are not the cause. The term Alzheimer's disease describes a pre-senile dementia, usually affecting patients aged 40–60 years. Histologically the brain resembles a senile one with marked cortical atrophy, neurofibrillary tangles and silver staining (senile) plaques. The cause is unknown.

Clinical features

There is a gradual onset of dementia which progresses affecting all intellectual and social functions. Symptoms include loss of memory for recent events, inability to reason and make good judgements, alterations of affect and emotional reactions, and sometimes the development of delusions. Later there may be loss of personal care and hygiene with incontinence. There will then also be physical deterioration often with the appearance of cortico-spinal and cortico-bulbar and extrapyramidal signs. In some patients epileptic seizures may appear. GPs will often notice increased irritability in such patients and a tendency to hypochondriasis in the early stages.

There is no effective treatment and many patients with early onset dementias survive for only 3 to 5 years from the time of diagnosis.

Multi-infarct dementia

This is five times less common. It is due to diffuse atheroma of cerebral arteries. The pathology consists of micro- and macro-infarcts unevenly distributed in the brain. Destruction of the more centrally placed temporal lobe grey matter is particularly associated with recent memory loss. This area is largely supplied from the posterior cerebral artery.

Clinical features

It is more common in men. The dementia may affect all functions but sometimes one particular one is lost to a more marked extent, e.g. memory. Emotional lability and irritability are often prominent. There may be an abrupt onset with a step-wise deterioration. Fluctuations may arise in the symptoms. Associated features – hypertension, coronary artery disease, fundal changes and a degree of 'Parkinsonism' may be present.

Overall prognosis of dementia

The outlook is variable but generally unfavourable. Unless there is a remedial cause no-one improves but in some patients progress may be very slow. Kay[21] showed that 75% were dead in four years compared with 26% of normal controls. The best prognostic indicator appeared to be poor memory when compared with age, physical disability, falls, poor living conditions and social isolation. Institutionalisation may hasten the progress of the disease or at least the effects of it. About 15% of demented patients are in institutions at any one time.

Normal pressure hydrocephalus *(NPH)*

NPH is a rare but important cause because it may be correctable. The cerebral ventricles enlarge following disturbance of the CSF circulation usually as a late result of infection, trauma or haemorrhage. It is possible there are problems in the formation and absorption of CSF, and it fails to pass over the surface of the brain. Signs of raised intracranial pressure are absent.

NPH presents as memory failure, with mental deterioration, unsteady gait with short shuffling steps, urinary incontinence and lack of insight with, sometimes, aggression.

Suspected patients will need neurological referral for scanning as ventriculo-atrial or peritoneal shunts may produce improvement in selected patients.

Looking for a cause

(1)   Check for any evidence of an acute confusional state – dehydration, infection, fatigue, malnutrition. The history from the patient and observers is crucial.

(2)   Assess the premorbid personality and behaviour from one's own memory, records, relatives and friends.

(3)   Seek evidence of mood change, emotional lability, use of alcohol, a history of trauma, falls or fits. Check any drugs prescribed.

(4)   Make due allowance for deafness, blindness, social isolation, language and cultural differences, previous known intelligence and level of social competence.

(5)   Examine verbally and physically for:

(a)   General appearance, nutrition, anaemia? myxoedema? uraemia? fever? tremor? injury? sobriety?

(b)   Infection, atheroma, heart disease, liver disease, carcinoma of bronchus.

(c) Is the patient depressed? Ask particularly about sleep patterns, diurnal variation of symptoms, previous mental health. Is the patient a schizophrenic?

(6) Assess higher functions and level of alertness:

(a) Assess memory loss.

Orientation in time and place.

Digit span – a normal adult can repeat back six digits.

Learning an eight word name and address or short sentence – normal adults can repeat back after two trials and recall it five minutes later.

Current events – allow for patient's interests and social isolation.

(b) Many patients with dominant hemisphere damage demonstrate a mixed dysphasia with difficulties in comprehension and expression. This may be associated with difficulties in reading, writing, in doing simple sums, in copying patterns and in word recognition. It may be possible to demonstrate the loss of ability to reason and solve problems but this may prove difficult and specialised psychological testing may be required.

Right hemisphere lesions are sometimes associated with difficulty in finding the way and with a disturbed body image so that a patient may not use a limb although he knows it is there (page 104).

(7) Decide:

(a) Is the patient dementing or merely confused? The latter will have a short history and there will usually be evidence of a recent cause.

(b) Is there need for referral – to obtain the specialist skills of a psychologist, psychiatrist, geriatrician, physician or neurologist. More information may be necessary from relatives, friends, social service workers or health visitors. A functional assessment may be obtained from social workers, occupational therapists or physiotherapists.

Investigations

Family doctors can organise a number of relevant investigations. These include:

A full blood count and ESR, serum B12 and folate levels, urea and electrolytes, liver function tests, thyroid function, WR or equivalent (to exclude syphilis).

The urine should be tested for sugar.

X-rays of the chest and skull.

At hospital a CT brain scan, EEG and other investigations may be undertaken.

Management

(1) As some 85% of patients show no remediable cause, the problem becomes one of functional assessment. Working with relatives, friends and associated health care professionals the family doctor must decide the degree of help the patient needs.

(2) Consider in turn – mobility, orientation, communication, restlessness, dressing, feeding, continence, sleep patterns and mood.

(3) Check correctable features – glasses, hearing aid, false teeth, anaemia, constipation, infection, etc. Treat depression if this is present.

(4) Consider the patients' insight into their problems and their wishes.

(5) Consider the degree of support available from relatives and friends. Social services may provide home help, meals-on-wheels, visits from health care workers, the district nurse, community psychiatric nurse and health visitor. Caring agencies include voluntary organisations, church and neighbourhood groups. Many patients end in residential homes or hospitals.

Medication

This has little place. Vasodilators have little proven worth. Depression, agitation and disturbed sleep patterns are amenable to treatment but will rely on the correct dose being given – often difficult to assess in the very old. Consider what arrangements can be made for this if it is necessary. Thioridazine (Melleril) may help some demented patients with disturbed behaviour and agitation. Haloperidol (Serenace) by intramuscular injection can be used in an emergency.

Relatives

It is important to involve the relatives at every step. Try and give a realistic picture of the prognosis and emphasise the value of keeping the patient in familiar surroundings as long as possible. Their wishes are important but the extent of the pressures upon them from other sources in their lives (finances, teenagers, marital strains, etc.) may not be known to the GP. Relatives may be concerned that the commitment to a dementing patient will leave them inadequately supported by other services. Give information about available resources as holiday relief, incontinence and laundry services, attendance at day centres, etc. Maintain a good relationship with the family and try to keep in touch regularly and with other members of the practice team. Regular review meetings with the team may prove helpful. In many patients at a later stage a decision may have to be made about long-term hospital placement.

Remember if there is any doubt about depression presenting as a pseudo-dementia, it is worth a trial of anti-depressant treatment.

8

Cerebrovascular Disease

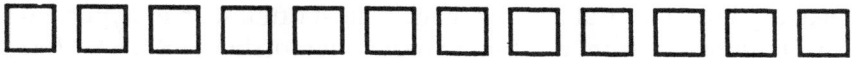

STROKES

Incidence

Strokes are common, with an incidence of between one and two per 1,000 of the population; these figures rising with increasing age. The GP with an average list of about 2,500 patients will expect to see some five new patients with strokes each year.

Types

Strokes are divided into thrombo-embolic infarcts (some 80%) and haemorrhagic infarcts (some 20%). About one half of the thrombo-embolic infarcts are due to emboli arising from the heart. Nearly three-quarters of stroke patients are admitted to hospital.

Outcome

Strokes carry a significant mortality; about one-third of patients have died within one month. Of the survivors, one-third recover, one-third remain disabled, and one-third are totally dependent.

Thus there is also an appreciable morbidity. Furthermore patients who have sustained a stroke are at greater risk from another episode. Of ultimate survivors about another 25–50 per cent will have further strokes[22].

Pathology

Patients who have sustained a completed stroke will show evidence of persisting neurological damage. This will depend on the site and extent of the neuronal loss. Haemorrhagic infarcts may arise from primary intracerebral haemorrhage – most often seen in hypertensive patients, or from a sub-arachnoid haemorrhage (SAH). Most SAHs are due to a ruptured aneurysm, a few from angiomas or bleeding disorders. In about 20% of patients with SAH who are investigated by angiography no cause is found. Emboli causing cerebral infarcts may arise from mural thrombus in the heart at the site of a myocardial infarct, or from diseased valves. Emboli may also arise from atheromatous damaged extracranial arteries. Thrombotic occlusion of diseased arteries, narrowed by atheroma, also occurs.

Presentation

Embolic infarcts usually have a sudden onset. Haemorrhagic strokes also have an acute onset, sometimes following physical exertion or emotion. Thrombotic infarcts may have a slower onset over some hours. Many strokes are first recognised on waking. Headache, vomiting and meningism are common with haemorrhage but about 15% of patients with intracerebral haemorrhage may show no meningism and no CSF xanthochromia. Extensive areas of damage or brain swelling will cause depression or loss of consciousness.

Signs

Most patients with strokes have weak or paralysed limbs. A hemisphere infarct may cause a hemiparesis. This may be accompanied by hemisensory loss, a hemianopia (in more posteriorly placed lesions) and dysphasia (page 104) if the dominant (usually left) hemisphere is damaged (Figure 21). These signs are contralateral to the damaged hemisphere in infarcts in the carotid artery territories. Initially paretic limbs may appear flaccid but within days become spastic with exaggerated reflexes and an extensor plantar response. Extensive infarcts producing a depressed conscious level may cause an irregular waxing and waning pattern of respiration, Cheyne–Stokes breathing. With major damage in the anterior part of the hemisphere there may be deviation of the eyes and head towards the damaged hemisphere and away from the paralysed limbs (pages 99 and 100).

Hind brain strokes

Vertebro-basilar (VB) territory damage may cause more extensive and varied signs, for in addition to the nuclei of the cranial nerves, the long tracts also pass through the brain stem. Usually hind brain damage causes ipsilateral cerebellar upset with often an ipsilateral Horner's syndrome. High up in the midbrain there are commonly visual movement disorders with involvement of the oculomotor nerve, in the pons facial sensory upset, facial weakness and abducens nerve involvement, and lower down in the brain stem deafness, vertigo, vomiting, hiccup and bulbar symptoms with dysphagia. Long tract involvement may produce pyramidal distribution weakness and spinothalamic sensory loss – these last signs may be contralateral. Posterior cerebral artery involvement is likely to produce a hemianopia.

Sub-arachnoid haemorrhage *(SAH)*

Patients present with the acute onset of severe headache (page 26) often accompanied by vomiting. The headache may be very severe and there may even be loss of consciousness. Some patients present with a fit. Some 10% of patients probably die immediately. The survivors show signs of meningism, photophobia, drowsiness and irritability. Occasionally patients may appear confused but a sudden onset with meningism should alert the doctor to the possibility of a bleed or meningitis. Patients may show focal signs as an oculomotor palsy or hemiparesis. There may be papilloedema or the presence of a subhyaloid haemorrhage. Sometimes back pain is prominent.

Course Patients require admission to hospital. There is a significant chance of rebleeding: about 50% of patients will die in the first three months from a further bleed. Identification of the source of bleeding by angiography may allow the surgical clipping of an aneurysm.

Primary intracerebral haemorrhage

Haemorrhagic strokes are more severe and carry a high mortality; some 80% of patients die. Such patients are often hypertensive and may have a very depressed conscious level. Relatively large areas of haemorrhage tend to occur in the basal ganglia, thalamus and brain stem. Supratentorial bleeds may cause a rapidly expanding lesion with coning. Hypertensive patients may rupture small micro-aneurysms (described by Charcot and Bouchard in 1868) which again appear concentrated in the striatum, thalamus and pons. These may produce small infarcts with much less upset.

Patients with haemorrhagic strokes commonly require admission to hospital.

In patients suspected of a stroke, ask:

(1) Is the diagnosis correct? About 5% of patients diagnosed as having a stroke have tumours or other pathology.

(2) If this is a stroke, has the patient reached their worst? A proportion of patients show an evolving picture with deterioration. This may be due to cerebral oedema, airway obstruc-

118

tion, the development of pneumonia or cardiac failure, further haemorrhage or that the original diagnosis was wrong.

(3) Can the family of the patient cope with such a patient at home? Admission may also be necessary because the first two questions cannot be answered. Often the patient's age, general medical state and home conditions strongly influence the decision about admission and about 75% of patients are admitted.

Home nursing

If patients are to be nursed at home, considerable support must be given and the family needs instructions. The community nurse may give these. She may also help with bathing, problems with bowel and bladder and provision of simple aids. Home physiotherapy and speech therapy, where appropriate and available, may also be of value. A home assessment visit from the occupational therapist of the local social services may allow provision of certain disabled aids in the home.

Investigations

Patients nursed at home may need some investigations. These are important in younger patients, who are at risk from further strokes.

(1) *Blood sample* Full blood count, packed cell volume and ESR. Urea, electrolytes, glucose. Younger patients add – lipid profile, thyroid function, Wassermann reaction.

(2) *ECG* Cardiac source from emboli?

(3) *Chest X–ray* (where feasible) Carcinoma lung, heart size?

In instances of diagnostic doubt further studies may be necessary and these require attendance at hospital.

Psychological Effects

In many patients a stroke may lead to loss of independence, and in younger patients the loss of their role as 'bread-winner' or 'mother' in the family. Many patients become depressed, some apathetic and such upsets need treatment, support and encouragement.

Some strokes, by their site, create problems with memory, changes in behaviour, personal neglect and even incontinence. Non–dominant hemisphere strokes may cause neglect of the affected limbs.

Active physiotherapy, occupational therapy, attendance at day centres or even participation in the activities of various social clubs may help.

Driving

This to some extent will depend on the patient's age and residual disability. Paralysed limbs, a hemianopia, severe dysphasia or inco-ordination may prove major handicaps. However, if a deficit is static and the patient has adapted to it then driving may be possible although sometimes special controls or automatic transmission may be necessary. Most patients after a major stroke should not drive for some twelve months if they have been left with deficits to which they have to adapt.

TRANSIENT ISCHAEMIC ATTACKS (TIAs)

Definition These are episodes, transient in duration, of focal neurological dysfunction usually lasting minutes and followed by full recovery. By definition if they last more than 24 hours or are followed by signs of residual damage then a completed stroke has occurred. Their importance is because they may herald a completed stroke. The incidence for this varies with different series but about one third of patients who present with TIAs have developed a completed stroke within five years.

Pathogenesis TIAs largely arise from fibrin–platelet emboli often originating from atheromatous damage in extracranial arteries. In some 30% the source is the heart – mural infarcts or valvular disease. Less commonly there may be drops in cerebral perfusion linked with changes in heart rate or rhythm, or a very high or low blood pressure. TIAs may also be precipitated by severe anaemia, polycythaemia, and by hypoglycaemia. They may also be provoked on a mechanical basis by head turning where atheromatous vertebral arteries are compromised in their passage through the cervical vertebrae.

Symptoms TIAs can be divided into carotid and vertebro-basilar (VB) territory episodes. They are more common in the VB territory but have a higher stroke risk in the carotid territory.

Carotid Territory

These include transient episodes of monocular visual loss, amaurosis fugax, where patients describe a 'shutter or blind' coming down over the field of vision. The loss is painless and there is full recovery within minutes. Such episodes are ipsilateral to the artery affected. TIAs involving the hemisphere produce symptoms contralateral to the side affected. These include weakness in the limbs, sometimes brachiofacial in distribution. Hemisensory changes may also occur and even speech upset with dysphasia if the dominant hemisphere is affected.

Vertebro-basilar Territory

These may cause dizziness with unsteadiness, vertigo and vomiting, visual upset (with diplopia or bilateral visual disturbance), drop attacks, facial sensory upset (often circumoral), and alternating hemipareses or hemisensory upsets (first one side then the other).

Signs

During an attack abnormal signs may be present and rarely emboli may be seen in a retinal vessel. However, most patients are seen between episodes and may show no abnormal signs. However, they may give a history of angina or claudication and a number have stigmata of vascular disease – bruits over neck vessels or the groins, hypertension, signs of heart disease, a blood pressure unequal in the two arms (suggesting a possible subclavian 'steal') or lost pedal pulses.

Rarely, focal fits from a tumour or other pathology as a subdural haematoma may present with TIAs.

Subclavian Steal

Stenosis of the proximal part of one subclavian artery may allow reversal of blood flow down the vertebral artery starving the brain stem and producing hind–brain ischaemia. This may be precipitated by exercising an arm. Such patients show an inequality of the radial pulses and blood pressure in the two arms, and often a bruit in the supraclavicular fossa.

Investigations of TIAs

Most younger patients will need hospital referral. However, GPs may often manage patients. They should:

(1) Take blood for a full blood count, PCV, ESR, lipid profile, glucose and Wassermann (or equivalent)
(2) Test urine for sugar and protein
(3) Arrange an ECG
(4) Arrange X–rays of the chest and skull.

Management of TIAs

There has been much recent discussion about the best treatment of TIA[23]. A very high blood pressure should be controlled (ideally bringing the diastolic pressure down to between 90–100 mm Hg): care must be taken in the elderly. Smokers are strongly encouraged to stop.

Surgery Carotid territory TIAs may arise from a local atheromatous lesion near the origin of the internal carotid artery – either a tight stenosis (often accompanied by a bruit) or a local shallow ulcer. Surgical disobliteration of this site may prevent further TIAs and strokes. However, angiography and surgery carry a mortality and morbidity (hopefully low) and if patients treated by successful surgery are followed, a proportion die from myocardial infarcts confirming that they have wide–spread arterial disease. This has led to increasing interest in medical treatment.

Anticoagulants The first medical treatment was warfarin (and other anticoagulants). These have been shown as beneficial in the first 6 to 12 months but with prolonged use the risks of bleeding are greater than those of developing a stroke[24]. Patients with a definite cardiac source of emboli should be treated with anticoagulants and these may be necessary long–term. Such patients require blood tests to monitor control.

Anti-platelet drugs. Aspirin at present holds the best outlook although this currently is under an extended trial. Low dose regular aspirin (the exact dose is uncertain – 300–1200 mg daily have been used) appears to reduce the risks of further strokes or TIAs in men under the age of 65[25]. In other patients the position at present is less definite. However treatment is easy and well tolerated unless patients show gastric intolerance to aspirin.

Other drugs have also been used. These include dipyridamole (Persantin) and sulphinpyrazone (Anturan). Dipyridamole and warfarin have been shown to reduce the incidence of emboli from prosthetic heart valves as compared to warfarin alone, but in another trial dipyridamole used alone did not prevent TIAs. In the authors' view sulphinpyrazone and dipyridamole are ineffective.

STROKE RISK FACTORS

Hypertension	systolic and diastolic
Cardiac Source	myocardial infarct, valvular disease, prosthetic valves, heart failure, arrhythmias, atrial fibrillation

High haematocrit

Smoking

Diabetes mellitus

High plasma lipids particularly men under the age of 55

Thyrotoxicosis

Oral contraceptive pill

Note about 25% of strokes are *preceded by a TIA.*

GP's Role in Prevention

Check blood pressure

Advise stop smoking

Search for diabetes – control of disease in known diabetics

Supervision of women on the contraceptive pill.

9

Back and Limb Pain, Weakness

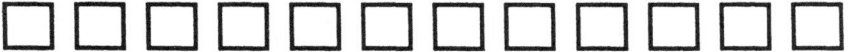

BACK PAIN

This is common in the neck and lumbar regions; the two sites of maximal spinal movement. Low back pain (LBP) is responsible for 6.5% of all GP consultations. The thoracic spine is splinted by the ribs and much less often is a site for pain. The spine is very strong: anteriorly it is formed by the vertebral bodies, separated by the discs which are supported by the anterior and posterior longitudinal ligaments. The spinal canal is formed by the pedicles, laminae and spinous and transverse processes at the sides and back which are largely supported by the strong paraspinal muscles (Figure 16). The spinal cord is shorter than the canal ending at the lower border of L1; below that the cauda equina carries the lumbosacral roots to the exit foramina from the canal. Lumbosacral disc protrusions compress the nerve roots below the cord termination, but cervical disc protrusions may compress both roots and the spinal cord.

Pain

Back and limb pains arise in many ways. They may be local from the bones, joints, ligaments or muscles commonly supplied by

Figure 16 Diagram of fourth lumbar vertebra seen from above
(1) Central disc protrusion compressing cauda equina
(2) Lateral disc protrusion compressing nerve root

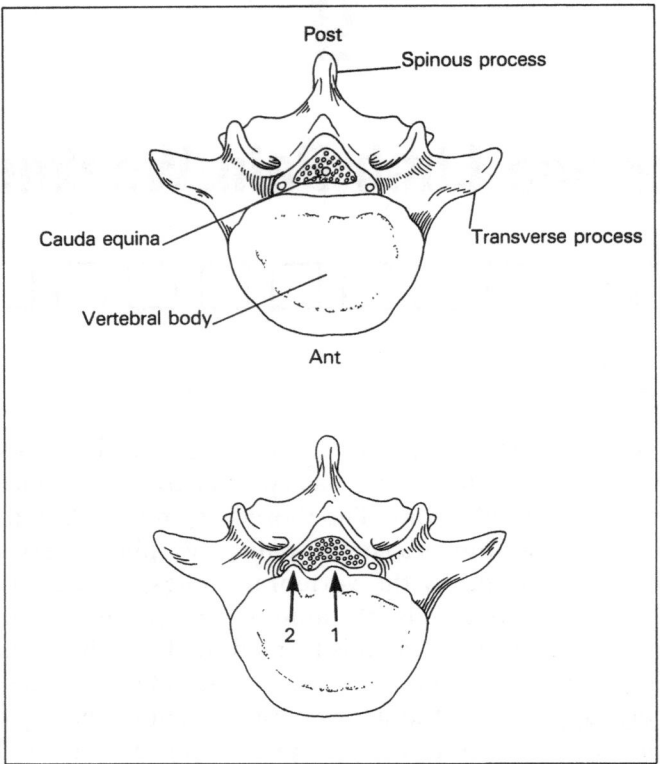

meningeal branches of the spinal nerves. Protective paraspinal muscle spasm is often prominent in neck and low back pain. Local back pain may also arise from the posterior annulus of the disc as it starts to bulge or 'slip'. If a nerve root is irritated this will usually produce pain radiating into the affected myotome (Figures 17 and 18). If the nerve is then compressed, there may be local weakness of muscles supplied by that root, a depressed or absent reflex at that level, and sensory symptoms with impaired sensation in the appropriate dermatome (Figures 17 and 18).

126

Figure 17(a) Sclerotome distribution of root pain
(b) Dermatome distribution of sensory symptoms

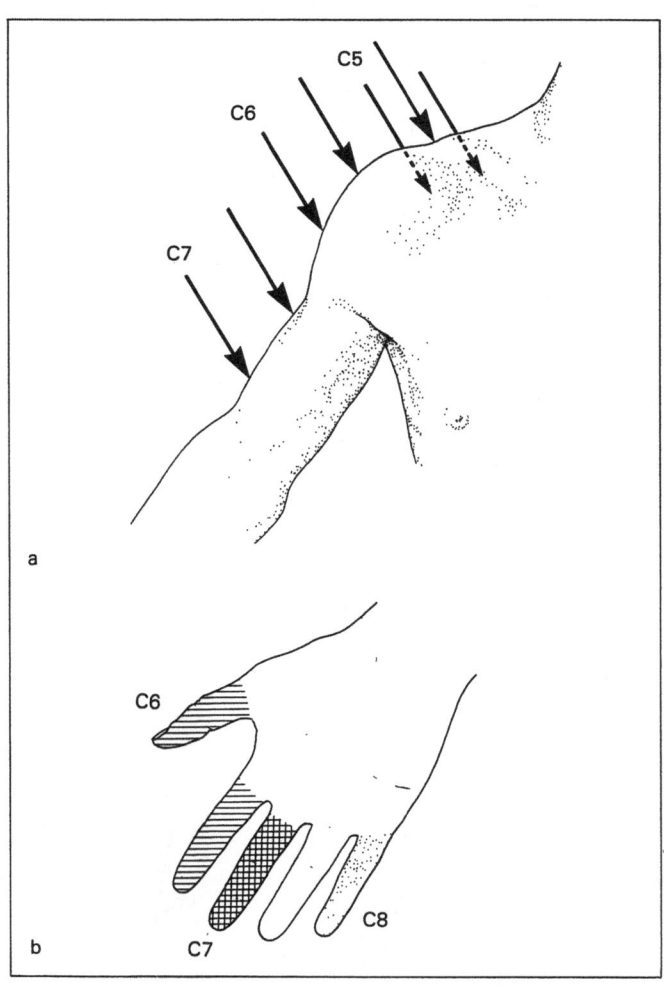

Figure 18(a) Sclerotome distribution of sciatica
(b) Dermatome distribution of sensory symptoms for L 5 and
S 1 roots

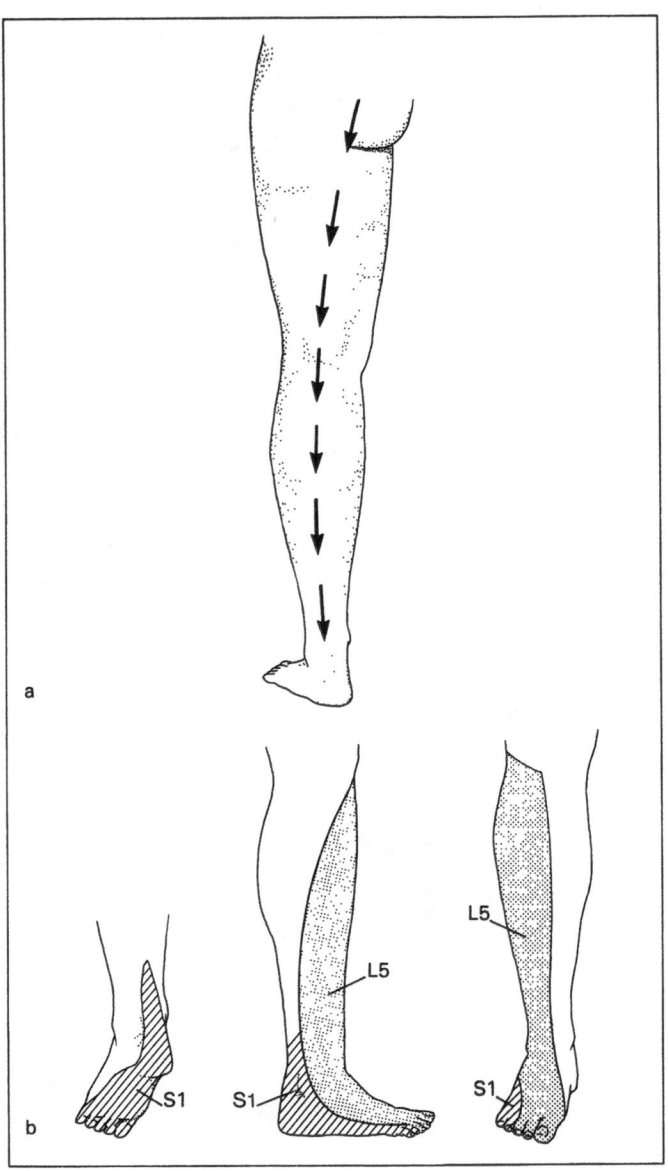

Referred pain

Pain may be referred in both directions. Root pain from irritation, inflammation, compression or stretching, may be referred to the limb or around the trunk. Conversely local structures, as diseased bowel or pelvic viscera, may present with pain referred to the back.

History

History is important, particularly the mode of onset, the site and duration of the pain, any reference, and any factors which aggravate or relieve this. Limb pains aggravated by coughing, sneezing, or exertion suggest root irritation. Most pain from disc prolapse is relieved by rest. Pain made worse lying, especially at night, suggests possible malignant disease. Pain may sometimes be aggravated by exercise and relieved by rest to a degree as to suggest claudication, either from arterial insufficiency or from a lumbar canal stenosis.

Weakness, loss of use or sensory symptoms strongly suggest nerve involvement and any account of sphincter disturbance should always be viewed seriously.

Examination of the spine

It is best to examine the spine and limbs in such patients without clothes which may obscure wasting or a scoliosis. In acute· disc protrusions all spinal or neck movements are limited. In lumbosacral lesions, forward trunk flexion is limited, and sometimes lateral flexion: straight leg raising is also limited often indicating that a nerve root is under tension.

Questions

The family doctor must ask:

(1)   Are the symptoms arising in the back or neck?

129

(2) If so, what is the cause?

(3) Are there signs to support root or peripheral nerve irritation or damage?

(4) If so, what is the pathogenesis?

(5) Is this a more generalised disturbance with widespread weakness or other signs?

Depending on the answers, the decision must be taken as to whether the patient needs hospital referral, or can be investigated and treated by the GP.

ARM PAIN AND WEAKNESS

Arm and neck pains are common, about 10% of the population complain of them at any one time. Other causes as joint disease, painful 'arcs' in the shoulder, 'tennis elbow', local injuries or even bone metastases may need exclusion.

Arm pain may arise *proximally* from *nerve root* involvement in:

(A) Cervical spine

(1) acute soft disc prolapse

(2) rough bone surfaces or spurs (osteophytes)

(3) disc degeneration with spondylosis – the most common cause

(4) other diseases (rare), e.g. neoplasia

(5) herpes zoster – this may cause acute root pain at any level but the rash will give the diagnosis.

Disc prolapse and spondylosis commonly cause:

Root irritation with pain referred to the appropriate sclerotome (Figure 17a) and sensory symptoms (Figure 17b). In order of decreasing frequency C 5/6 (C6 root), C 6/7 (C7 root), C 4/5 (C5 root) and C 3/4 (C 4 root) are the levels most affected.

Root compression with weakness, sensory signs and reflex changes at the appropriate level (Figure 1, Tables 3 and 4).

130

Root and spinal cord involvement, with a combination of signs in the arms from root damage, a radiculopathy, and signs in the legs from cord involvement, a myelopathy. In the legs there is usually spastic weakness with exaggerated reflexes and extensor plantar responses. These may be accompanied by sensory changes particularly posterior column sensory loss and sometimes by sphincter upset (urgency and frequency of micturition and constipation). High cervical cord lesions, above C 4, may cause severe postural loss in the fingers. *X-rays* of the cervical spine may confirm the diagnosis. A lateral canal diameter of <10 mm suggests that the cord is compressed.

(B) Brachial plexus

(a) Acute inflammatory upset, *neuralgic amyotrophy*, presents with intense pain in the shoulder and arm followed by the development of weakness, wasting and reflex changes. Sometimes there may be sensory changes and the condition may be bilateral. Given time most patients recover spontaneously.

(b) *Malignant infiltration* – most often from breast or lung cancer. This causes progressive painful weakness and wasting, sometimes accompanied by marked swelling of the arm (particularly after a mastectomy), with sensory symptoms and reflex depression or loss.

(c) *Fibrosis of the plexus* usually starting 6–18 months after radio–therapy for breast cancer. Commonly presents with painless progressive weakness.

(C) Peripheral nerve

Common entrapment sites are:

Carpal tunnel The median nerve is compressed in the carpal tunnel at the wrist. Commonly this presents with painful tingling awakening patients at night. Women are more often affected. Later there may be weakness with wasting of the thenar muscles

131

and sensory impairment in the median three and a half fingers (Figure 19). There may be complaints of pain, sometimes referred up the arm, and aggravated by use. The carpal tunnel syndrome is sometimes symptomatic of diabetes, myxoedema, or rheumatoid arthritis: it may also arise in pregnancy. EMG studies will confirm the diagnosis.

Treatment In mild cases there may be relief by sleeping in a wrist splint or by local steroid injection. In more severe cases surgical decompression is necessary.

The ulnar nerve at the elbow An ulnar palsy may present with tingling and numbness in the little and ring fingers (Figure 19) and/or with weakness and wasting of the small hand muscles (interossei) and hypothenar muscles which causes loss of facility for fine manipulative movements. The thenar pad muscles are spared. Sometimes the ulnar nerve is obviously thickened at the elbow and there may be deformity at that site from past injury. Most patients require hospital referral with a view to nerve conduction studies. Decompression of a site of local entrapment may afford relief and prevent deterioration but will seldom reverse any significant degree of muscle wasting, even if the nerve is also transposed.

LEG PAIN AND WEAKNESS

In the United Kingdom two million patients consult their GPs each year with low back pain. In some 80% this is non-specific with no particular cause but it may be accompanied by sciatica, referred pain from proximal root irritation most often due to a prolapsed intervertebral disc (PID). In others trauma, infection (e.g. TB), inflammation (ankylosing spondylitis), metabolic bone disease (with vertebral body compression) or metastases in bone, may be responsible.

132

Figure 19 The usual areas of sensory upset in lesions of the median, ulnar and radial nerves are shaded

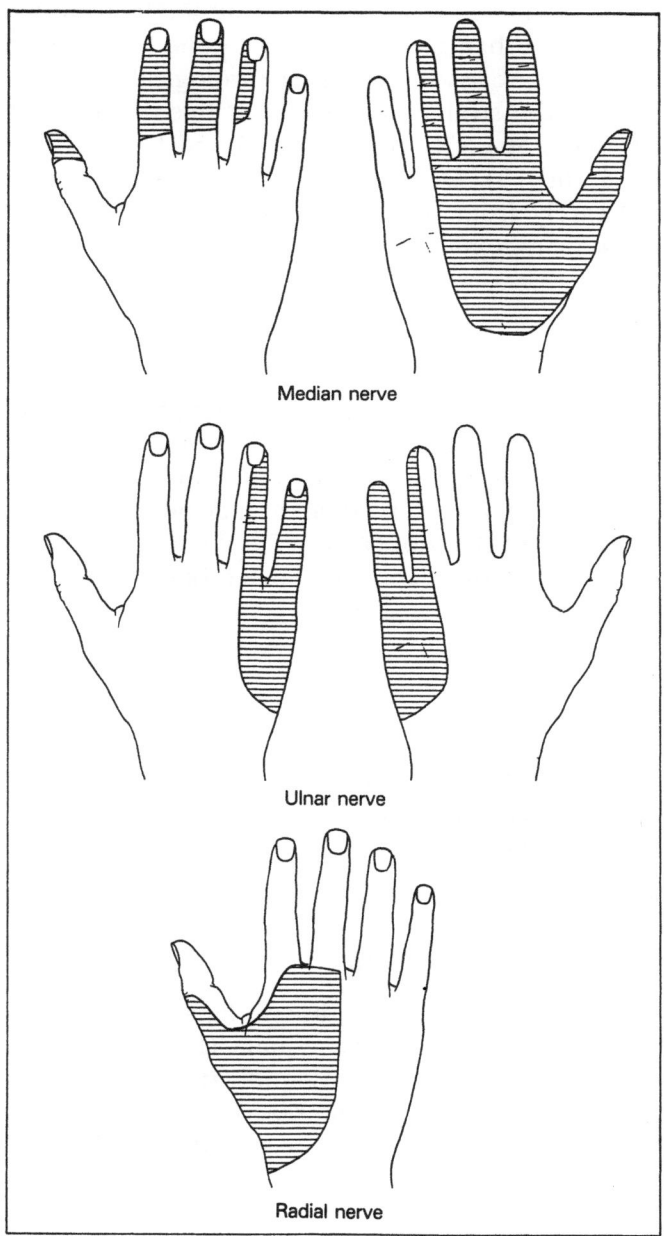

Median nerve

Ulnar nerve

Radial nerve

(A) Lumbosacral root involvement

This commonly follows some mechanical upset. Pain and weakness with sensory disturbances may appear in one leg often with low back pain. These are associated with neurological and root tension signs with reduced straight leg raising. If this is due to a PID, in 95% this occurs at L5/S1 (the S1 root) and L4/5 (the L5 root) (Figures 16 and 18). Damage may also occur from osteophytic spurs and rarely from other pathology – tumours, metastases, abscesses or lymphomas.

Signs

S1 damage will cause weakness standing on tiptoe on one foot with a lost ankle jerk. There may be sensory loss on the sole. L5 damage will produce weakness of extensor hallucis longus (sometimes the ankle dorsiflexors), a preserved ankle jerk but often sensory loss over the dorsum of the foot (Figure 2). Weakness of knee extension (quadriceps) with a depressed knee jerk suggests L3/4 disturbance (Tables 3 and 4).

Foot drop

This may arise from a PID, a lateral popliteal palsy or even a sciatic nerve lesion. It may also be part of a more generalised upset, e.g. peripheral neuropathy.

Bladder and bowel symptoms

These may arise acutely from a disc prolapse, particularly a large central protrusion in the cauda equina (Figure 16). This is an *emergency* for if the roots are not rapidly decompressed, irreversible damage to the control of the bladder and bowel may occur. Patients with these symptoms require urgent admission to hospital.

Treatment of the PID

Acute LBP with sciatica requires strict bed rest. This should be lying flat on a firm mattress or a bed with a board between the mattress and the springs (only getting up for bathroom purposes). Simple analgesics as aspirin, or paracetamol, or NSAIs as naproxen (Naprosyn) should be given regularly together with a muscle relaxant, as diazepam 5 mg b.d. and 10 mg nocte. As the acute pain subsides, it is usually possible to mobilise. Patients need instructions about the best position for lifting, and may benefit from exercises to strengthen the paraspinal muscles. With back pain some patients claim good relief by manipulation but this should be avoided if there is any diagnostic doubt or any signs or symptoms of nerve involvement.

Pain persists – if this occurs doctors should arrange:

(1) Rectal and/or pelvic examination.
(2) Blood sample for full blood count, ESR, calcium, phosphatases, serum proteins and electrophoresis, and blood glucose.
(3) Urine sample for glucose, microscopy and culture.
(4) X-rays of the chest and appropriate part of the spine.

If there is a failure to respond to rest, repeated incapacitating attacks of pain or progressive neurological deficit, patients should be referred to hospital. Surgical excision of a PID is necessary in about 10%.

(B) Diabetic amyotrophy

Diabetes may produce an acute vasculitis of the vasa nervorum producing painful peripheral nerve damage, most commonly seen in the femoral nerve. Patients present with severe pain in the thigh, often worse at night, associated with weakness and wasting of the quadriceps muscle and loss of the knee jerk. In most patients there are also signs to suggest the presence of a more widespread crural neuropathy – lost ankle jerks and impaired vibration sense in the feet. Pain in the leg may be the presentation of diabetes so all patients should have a urine sample tested. Most patients need hospital referral.

(C) Lateral cutaneous nerve of the thigh

Compression or irritation of this nerve where it passes under the inguinal ligament just medial to the anterior superior iliac spine may produce pain, tingling or numbness in an area, about the size of a hand, on the anterolateral aspect of the thigh – *meralgia paraesthetica*. It may be provoked by weight gain, pregnancy or found in diabetics. Usually reassurance and time are all that are necessary. Rarely discomfort is so bad that surgical exploration is necessary.

(D) Lateral popliteal (common peroneal) nerve palsy

Damage to this nerve is most often produced by compression at the head of the fibula: rarely it may be compressed here by a ganglion, neuroma or a tendinous band – most often by external pressure. The presentation is with a foot drop with weakness of the toe and ankle dorsiflexors and evertors. The ankle jerk is commonly preserved and there is no weakness of the hamstrings which may help to differentiate it from an L5/S1 root lesion. The area of sensory loss is very similar to that of an L5 root lesion (Figure 20). EMG studies will aid the diagnosis and referral is usually necessary.

GENERALISED WEAKNESS

This may arise from:
(1) Peripheral neuropathy – here there is commonly distal weakness with depressed or absent reflexes and sensory symptoms or loss.

Figure 20 The usual areas of sensory upset in lesions of the lateral popliteal and sciatic nerves are shaded

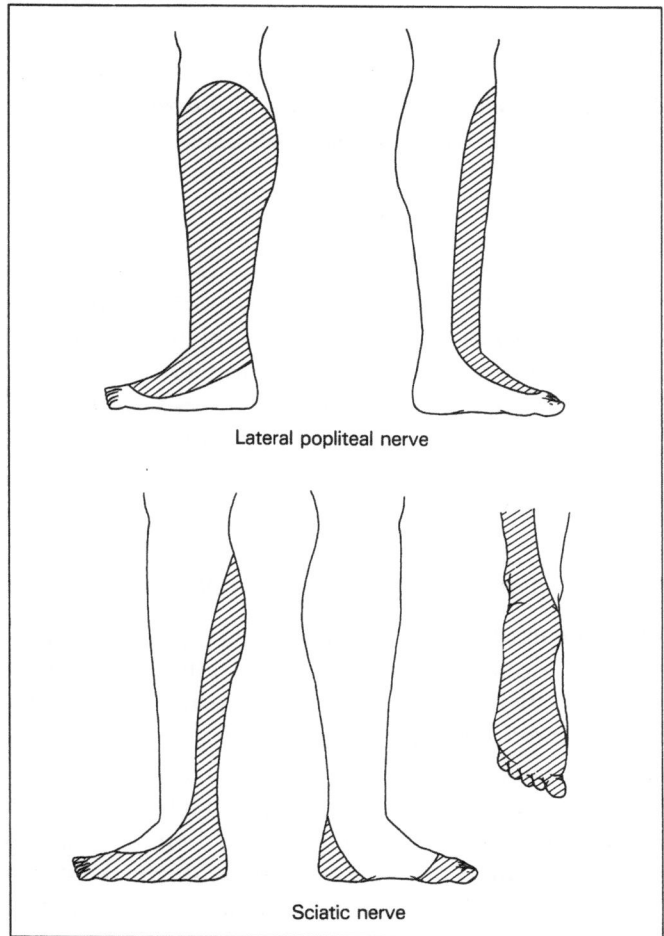

(2) Myopathy – most often seen with weakness of proximal muscles.

(3) Muscle fatiguability – as seen in myasthenia gravis where the presentation is often with ocular or bulbar symptoms. These may fluctuate.

(4) Systemic disease – as hypokalaemia, Addison's disease or malignancy.

(5) Functional complaints – often reflecting anxiety and/or depression.

Check Any family history of neuromuscular upset and whether the patient is taking any drugs or toxic substances.

Polyneuritis

This may arise acutely as in the Guillain–Barré syndrome – acute polyneuropathy, or more slowly. Damage may occur to the myelin sheath, the cell body or its process, the axon. Often it is mixed. The *acute inflammatory polyneuropathy* illustrates well the features of a polyneuritis. In some 50% there is a preceding history of a respiratory or gastrointestinal infection.

Symptoms and signs of acute inflammatory polyneuropathy

Weakness is the major symptom spreading rapidly over a period of days. Although commonly this starts distally in the legs, it then spreads proximally and may involve arm, trunk and facial muscles – the last in some 50%. The *bulbar muscles* may be affected with problems in swallowing and speaking in some 30%, and the *respiratory muscles* become severely affected in some 25%. Respiratory failure unless recognised and treated may prove fatal. In many patients pain is prominent, often in the back, attributed to acute inflammation of the nerve roots. *Sensory symptoms* are often less striking but may include distal tingling, numbness and sensations of walking on wool. The sensory upset may spread into a long glove–stocking distribution. *Autonomic nerves* may be involved causing postural hypotension, disorders of heart rate, urinary retention, loss of sweating and constipation.

Course

In over 90% the disease has reached its worst by 10 – 14 days and most patients will eventually make a good recovery. Rarely acute porphyria may present in this way.

Reflexes

In addition to prominent weakness patients show depressed or absent reflexes.

Cranial nerves

These may be involved, particularly the facial nerves. Mild bilateral facial weakness may be missed as the face appears symmetrical. Bulbar weakness must be recognised as this may lead to aspiration pneumonia.

Management

If the diagnosis is suspected, patients must be admitted to hospital in view of the possibility of progression to life-threatening respiratory or bulbar complications. The condition is usually self-limiting.

Chronic polyneuropathy

More chronic forms of neuropathy arise from numerous causes; in nearly a half no cause is identified. The most common causes are:

(1) Diabetes mellitus.
(2) An occult carcinoma, most commonly of the lung, but also lymphomas.
(3) Vitamin B12 deficiency.

(4) Drugs – nitrofurantoin (Furadantin), isoniazid (Rimifon), vincristine (Oncovin) or toxic substances as alcohol, lead or gold.

Many other causes may be responsible. Leprosy is still one of the most common causes in the world. Patchy nerve damage from involvement of the blood supply to peripheral nerves may occur in connective tissue disorders as polyarteritis nodosa, rheumatoid arthritis, systemic lupus erythematosus. This may also occur in diabetes and in sarcoidosis. Such patchy damage may involve several different peripheral nerves in an asymmetrical fashion – a *mononeuritis multiplex*. Deficiency states as in malnutrition and vitamin B1 deficiency may cause a neuropathy often with marked sensory symptoms – 'burning feet'. These symptoms also occur in diabetic and alcoholic neuropathy.

Rare *heredo-familial forms* may appear. The family history is important and there may be dominant inheritance as in peroneal muscular atrophy (Charcot–Marie–Tooth disease). Such patients often have longstanding problems with distal weakness and wasting, associated with skeletal deformities and high arched feet, tight heel cords, trophic skin changes and even neuropathic joints (painless swollen disorganised joints). The peripheral nerves may be thickened.

Most patients require referral for investigation. GPs may arrange blood tests to exclude the most common causes. These include:

(1) Full blood count and ESR.

(2) Fasting blood glucose and two hour post-prandial sample.

(3) Serum B12 level.

(4) Chest X-ray.

Diabetic neuropathy

Most commonly this is a distal sensorimotor disturbance with weakness and often unpleasant sensory upset. Patients show distal weakness, absent ankle jerks and lost vibration sense in the feet. The legs are usually affected first but the hands may follow.

Diabetes may also produce an autonomic neuropathy with postural hypotension, sweating upsets, impotence, micturition disorders and nocturnal diarrhoea.

A mononeuropathy may occur with involvement of peripheral nerves, e.g. the femoral nerve (diabetic amyotrophy, page 135) and cranial nerves, e.g. the oculomotor nerve. These are often painful palsies. Patients with diabetes and mild neuropathic signs are more liable to develop nerve entrapment, e.g. carpal tunnel syndrome.

In all instances the best control of the diabetes is essential. A change to insulin may even be necessary.

MUSCLE DISEASE

This commonly affects proximal muscles. In the legs such weakness causes difficulties climbing stairs, getting out of a low chair or off the ground and in running. In the arms proximal weakness causes problems working above the head, brushing hair or putting on make-up. The muscle weakness is often associated with wasting, cramps and even pain. Reflexes are usually depressed or lost. Later in the illness affected muscles show contractures with fibrosis. Sensation is spared. Heart muscle may also be involved leading to ECG changes. Myotonia – delay in relaxation – is seen in myotonic dystrophy.

Myopathies include the *dystrophies*, inherited forms of muscle disease. Here accurate diagnosis is important to give a prognosis and genetic counselling. Many forms start in childhood. The most common is Duchenne which is X-linked affecting males, about one in 5,000 male births. This causes loss of the ability to walk by the age of 8 – 12 years and usually death in the late 'teens or early twenties.

Children present with delay in their motor milestones, often being slow to walk (after the age of 18 months), run, climb and hop. They may seem clumsy tending to fall frequently and their

141

speech may be delayed. They walk with a waddling gait with an excess lumbar lordosis from trunk and hip muscle weakness. Contractures of the heel cords may cause toe-walking.

Estimation of the muscle enzyme, *creatine kinase* (CK), is valuable as this will show a 30 – 300 fold increase. It will also be mildly elevated in most carriers of the disease (females). The CK is elevated in many forms of primary muscle disease with very high values in polymyositis. Other diseases which cause extensive muscle damage and even a myocardial infarct may cause a rise in CK.

Polymyositis

This is an acute inflammatory disease of muscle most often seen in adults aged 30 – 60, a little more common in women. Proximal muscles and those of the neck and bulb (speech and swallow) are most commonly involved. In 30 – 50% there is evidence of a connective tissue disorder, e.g. rheumatoid arthritis, systemic lupus erythematosus, and about 15% have an associated carcinoma. A dermatomyositis may also arise with associated skin changes; often a purplish rash over the face.

Hospital referral is necessary. An elevated CK may support the diagnosis. Patients are treated with steroids and often immuno suppressants.

There is also a childhood form of polymyositis.

Polymyalgia rheumatica

This presents in older patients (older than 50) with stiffness and pain in proximal muscles often worse on waking. There may be systemic upset with malaise, weight loss, a low fever and the ESR is usually more than 50 mm/hour. Many patients may develop a giant cell arteritis (page 28).

Treatment with prednisolone 20 – 30 mg daily will control the symptoms of polymyalgia. However, most patients will require a small maintenance dose of steroids for 6 – 24 months, a few even longer.

Drugs

Certain drugs may produce muscle weakness. The most common drug causes of a chronic proximal myopathy are from steroids, chloroquine (Avloclor, Nivaquine) and propranolol (Inderal). Alcohol may provoke an acute myopathy and hydralazine (Apresoline) a myositis. Pencillamine (Distamine) may produce myasthenia.

Muscle weakness also appears in:

(1) *Thyrotoxicosis.*

(2) *Hypokalaemia.*

Check the patient's serum thyroxine and potassium.

Myasthenia gravis

This is an uncommon disorder with an incidence of one per 10–20,000 causing excessive fatiguability in muscles from a fault at the neuromuscular junction. Modern studies suggest that this is an auto-immune disorder with the appearance of anti-acetylcholine receptor antibodies (found in some 90% of patients) which block the neurotransmitter, acetylcholine. This is released from nerve endings and cannot reach the active receptor site on the muscle folds.

Symptoms

Patients most often present with ocular symptoms – fatiguable ptosis and variable diplopia in 90%. They may be associated with facial and bulbar muscle weakness. There is commonly weakness of the neck, trunk and proximal limb muscles, particularly the triceps. Respiratory muscles may be involved. Patients may be misdiagnosed as functional, as when they are examined no signs

143

may be found. Re-examination in the evening or after exercise may be helpful.

Diagnosis

This can be confirmed by an edrophonium (Tensilon) test (page 96), EMG studies and estimation of anti-acetylcholine receptor antibody.

Management

Hospital referral will be necessary. Most patients are treated by anti-cholinesterases, neostigmine (Prostigmin) or pyridostigmine (Mestinon). Thymectomy, steroids and plasmapheresis together with immunosuppression may also be used in hospital.

The mainstay of treatment is the use of the anti-cholinesterases, neostigmine and pyridostigmine. A 15 mg tablet of neostigmine is equivalent to a 60 mg tablet of pyridostigmine. Diagnosed patients will usually be taking pyridostigmine regularly, often every 6 hours. Pyridostigmine has a longer duration of action, more even effect and less side effects.

Myasthenic patients on treatment may become weak from underdosage and this may become severe – a *myasthenic crisis* – with even life-threatening bulbar and respiratory difficulties. Such patients may need urgent hospital referral. This deterioration may be triggered by an acute infection.

Conversely patients may also become weak from overdosage of anti-cholinesterases – a *cholinergic crisis*. Here further tablets will make the weakness worse. An edrophonium (Tensilon) test will differentiate between the two. Edrophonium will make patients in a myasthenic crisis improve, but in a cholinergic crisis worse.

Myasthenic patients should not be started on steroids unless an in-patient as some patients may transiently deteriorate as treatment begins.

10

Gait Disorders

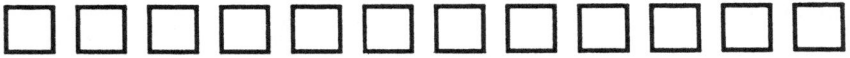

CAUSES

Many structures or systems may be at fault. The patient's age is important. Gait may be modified by:

Pain

(1) Local – infection or inflammation, e.g. infected corn, plantar fasciitis.

(2) Joints – infected or inflamed, e.g. rheumatoid arthritis, gout.

(3) Joints – degenerative changes, e.g. osteoarthritis hips, knees.

(4) Trauma – soft tissues, ligaments, bones.

(5) Bone disease

     Local – calcaneal spur

     Spinal – malignancy, infection, osteoporosis.

(6) Sciatica – referred spinal root pain (page 128)

(7) Vascular – claudication, phlebitis, ischaemia.

(8) Muscular – strain damage, inflammation, tendon rupture.

Mechanical

(1) Limbs of different length
        missed congenital hip dislocation.

(2) Restricted joint movements – degenerative or inflammatory
        loose bodies, torn cartilage, ankylosing spondylitis

Balance disturbances

Patients appear unsteady, may stagger or walk with a wide base
(page 63).

Extra pyramidal disorders (Parkinsonism)

Patients usually walk with short, shuffling steps with a flexed
posture, tending to festinate (hurry). The arms do not swing
(Chapter 13).

WEAKNESS IN CHILDREN

In the very young, delay in walking may indicate the possibility of a
number of disorders, many of neurological origin. Most children
start to walk between the ages of 12 – 16 months and are climbing
and running by the age of two. Any child that is not walking
unsupported by the age of 18 months needs to be examined and a
blood sample taken for a creatine kinase level. If the last is elevated, a muscular dystrophy needs consideration. It is important to
examine children naked so that the trunk, spine and limbs can be
fully viewed.

Spastic weakness, UMN problems

Such children may have a hemiplegia, diplegia (double hemiplegia) or paraplegia (legs alone). In the very young (in the first

twelve months of life) many children with spastic weakness appear 'floppy' with delayed motor milestones.

With an *infantile hemiplegia*, the affected limbs appear thinner, smaller and sometimes shorter. The reflexes are increased and the tone may be increased. A spastic diplegia may produce scissoring of the legs which appear stiff, often rather extended. There may be evidence of contractures as tight heel cords. Patients with only mild spastic weakness will have difficulty hopping or running. In attempting to walk on their heels or the outside of the feet (Fog's test), the hands and arms may go into odd positions. Abnormal arm and hand postures may also appear if the arms are held outstretched and supine or extended above the head. Minor asymmetries may suggest a UMN disturbance on the affected side.

Spastic children often show other abnormalities as choreo-athetosis, slurring dysarthria or even skeletal abnormalities.

Flaccid weakness, LMN problems

The anterior horn cell, peripheral nerve and muscle may be involved. Again there is a delay in motor milestones and 'floppiness'.

Proximal weakness will cause difficulty arising from a squatting position, in climbing tall steps or getting up from the ground. Such children may climb up themselves, using their arms to push on the legs to get the trunk upright (Gowers' sign). The gait may appear waddling with an exaggerated lumbar lordosis and protuberant abdomen from trunk muscle weakness, particularly seen in dystrophies.

Distal weakness is shown by problems walking on tiptoe or the heels. The feet may 'slap' and have to be lifted high from a foot drop. There is a tendency to trip. Wasted weak limbs are still seen as the residua of polio.

Some of these childhood disorders may be associated with tight heel cords, other muscle contractures, skeletal changes, e.g pes cavus, or developmental changes, e.g. talipes.

Sensory changes in the feet, lost reflexes, thickened peripheral nerves and painless swollen disorganised joints (neuropathic) suggest peripheral nerve involvement.

Conditions to be considered include:

(1) Anterior horn cells   spinal muscular atrophy.

(2) Peripheral nerves   often heredo-familial neuropathy (page 136).

(3) Muscles   dystrophies and polymyositis (page 142).

(4) Spinal dysraphism   malformations of the spine with involvement of the spinal cord and nerve roots.

These may be associated with deformities of the feet, a wasted leg, talipes, lost ankle jerks, occasionally an extensor plantar response and persistent incontinence. Nearly all children show some abnormality of the skin over the lumbosacral spine, often a hairy patch (faun's tail) or vascular naevus.

Fatiguable muscles

Childhood myasthenia is the most important. This most commonly starts in the external ocular muscles and may involve the face and bulbar muscles. Walking difficulties may appear. Myasthenia is discussed on page 143.

Weak muscles may also arise from primary muscle disease or in neurogenic damage and these may tire more quickly after exercise.

Clumsy, unsteady gait, often with weakness

This may arise from an acute cerebellar disturbance as from:

(1) Drug intoxication, e.g. phenytoin.

(2) Infections – often viral exanthemata or glandular fever.

148

More chronic problems may arise from:

(1) Developmental abnormalities often at the cranio-cervical junction, e.g. cerebellar ectopia, Chiari malformation.

(2) Posterior fossa tumours (page 72).

(3) Spino-cerebellar degenerations as *Friedreich's ataxia*. This is an inherited disorder, some dominant and some recessive, usually presenting with an unsteady gait between the ages of 10 – 20. There is difficulty standing and running. Later the hands become clumsy and the speech dysarthric.

Many show other skeletal abnormalities as scoliosis, pes cavus, clawed toes. Patients are ataxic showing Rombergism (more unsteady with the eyes closed). They have thin legs with absent reflexes and extensor plantar responses. Posterior column sensation is always upset (vibration and joint position). Nystagmus may or may not be present.

Diabetes is common and many patients show an abnormal ECG. The last is sometimes linked with the cause of an early death. Patients slowly deteriorate, often being confined to a wheelchair by the ages of 30 – 40, and many die early. There is no specific treatment.

General appearance

The appearance of the child is always important. General features, e.g. Mongolism or an extensive facial angioma (Sturge–Weber's syndrome), may give the diagnosis. Children with any form of mental retardation may show most unusual gaits.

In all these childhood conditions hospital referral will be necessary.

WEAKNESS IN ADULTS

Spastic weakness, UMN problems

This usually follows damage to the cortico-spinal tract

In the hemisphere (Figure 21)

Commonly this follows a stroke, less often after trauma, an infection or from a tumour. Spastic weakness appears in the contralateral leg which tends to drag, the foot being plantar-flexed and inverted. The whole leg appears stiff, extended and may circumduct while walking. The toe and outside edge of the shoe are often excessively worn. Repetitive rapid movements or hurrying are poorly performed.

A *parasagittal lesion* affecting the cortical motor areas for the legs in both hemispheres, as a meningioma, may produce a spastic paraparesis.

The medial part of the anterior three quarters of each cerebral hemisphere is supplied by the *anterior cerebral artery* (Figure 21). In some patients due to an anatomical variant, both hemispheres may be supplied by one anterior cerebral artery. A stroke in the territory of this vessel will cause a paraplegia with incontinence and *dysphasia*.

A thrombotic occlusion of one anterior cerebral artery (distal to Heubner's artery) may produce a flaccid weakness of the contralateral leg with exaggerated reflexes and an extensor plantar response. There may also be incontinence.

Patients with diffuse *frontal lobe damage* may show a marked gait disturbance walking with small shuffling steps in an uncertain fashion. They may show difficulty turning and starting movement yet appear to have relatively good leg movements when these are tested on the bed. This disorder is considered as an *apraxia of gait*. Patients with normal pressure hydrocephalus may show dementia, incontinence and a somewhat similar gait difficulty.

The cortico-spinal tracts may also be involved in their pathway down through the brain stem. Here damage usually produces other signs of cranial nerve and cerebellar involvement, and sometimes a Horner's syndrome.

150

Figure 21

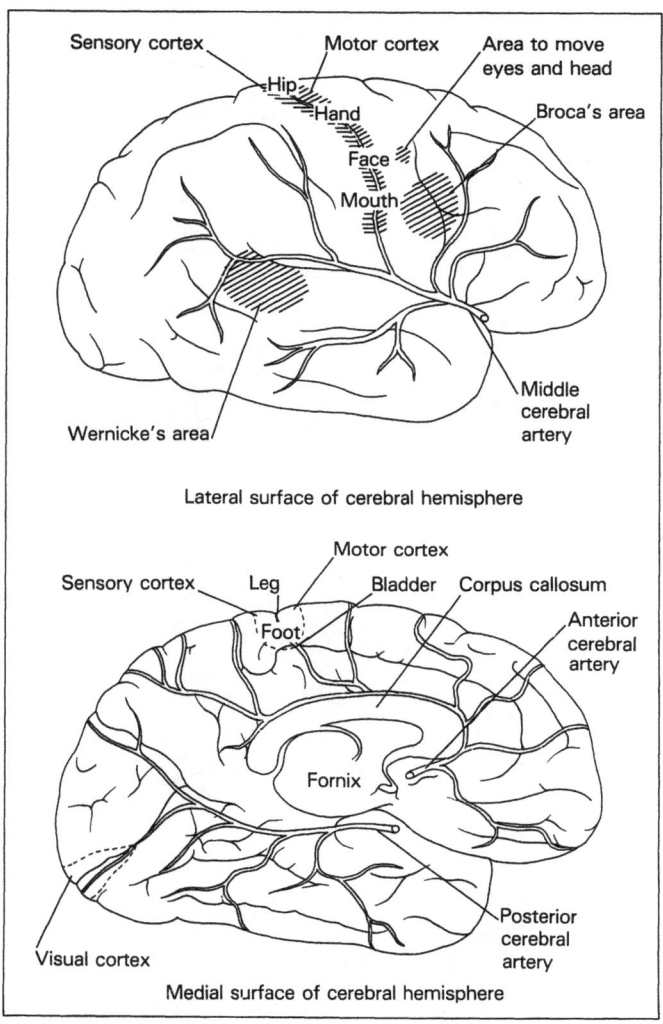

Lateral surface of cerebral hemisphere

Medial surface of cerebral hemisphere

Figure 22 Transverse sections of the spinal cord to show
(a) normal anatomy of the tracts
(b) site of a syrinx
(c) common sites for plaques in multiple sclerosis

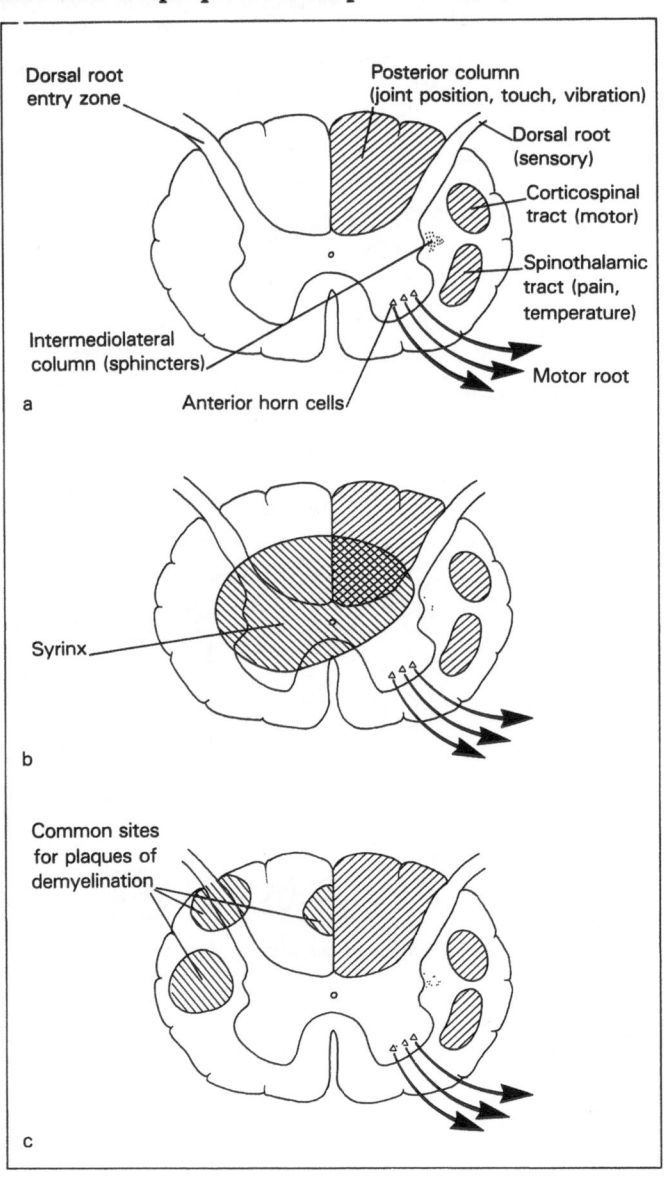

In the spinal cord (Figure 22)

A spastic paraparesis affects both legs producing a rather stiff slow gait with short steps, sometimes likened to someone wading through treacle. There may be adduction of the thighs and the toes may drag.

Spinal cord lesions may arise from:

(1) Compression by

    (a) Cervical spondylosis (page 30).

    (b) Spinal tumours (page 158).

    (c) Abscesses.

    (d) Trauma.

    (e) Others, e.g. skeletal deformities, haemorrhage.

(2) Inflammation by
    (a) Acute viral infection, e.g. zoster, polio post-vaccination.

    (b) Bacterial infection, e.g. tuberculosis, syphilis (rare).

    (c) Multiple sclerosis often a 'myelitis'.

(3) Metabolic upset e.g. sub-acute combined degeneration (page 155).

(4) Degeneration
    (a) Syringomyelia (page 155).

    (b) Spino-cerebellar degeneration, e.g. Friedreich's ataxia (page 149).

    (c) Familial spastic paraplegia.

    (d) Motor neurone disease (page 156).

(5) Vascular infarction (page 155).

Flaccid weakness, LMN problems

These are somewhat similar in distribution anatomically to those found in children although the causes may have a different emphasis. LMN weakness in the leg or legs may arise from damage to:

(1) Anterior horn cells	motor neurone disease, polio, spinal muscular atrophy.
(2) Peripheral nerves	neuropathies (page 136), particularly diabetes, drug-induced and non-metastatic carcinomatous types.
(3) Muscles	myopathies, dystrophies (page 141), thyrotoxicosis.

Associated with the weakness and sometimes separate from it, patients may show a *sensory ataxia* with loss of position sense in the toes and feet. This causes unsteadiness, which is worse in the dark or with the eyes closed (Rombergism). It is seen in tabes dorsalis (locomotor ataxia), diabetes, sub-acute combined degeneration, some spino-cerebellar degenerations and in some patients recovering after a severe acute Guillain–Barré polyneuritis. Such patients show marked loss of vibration and position sense in the feet, associated with reflex loss in the legs.

It is always worth checking a blood sample for:

(1) Blood glucose, preferably fasting and two hour postprandial.

(2) Wassermann (WR) or equivalent.

(3) Serum B12 level.

(4) Serum creatine kinase.

Fatiguable muscles

Myasthenia gravis (page 143).

SPINAL CORD INFARCTION

This is uncommon compared to the incidence of cerebral infarction. Usually the anterior spinal artery is involved. The onset is sudden, often over 1 to 2 hours, with bilateral leg weakness and dissociated sensory loss (spinothalamic loss with preservation of posterior column modalities) accompanied by loss of control of the bowel and bladder (Figure 22). The posterior spinal artery supplies the posterior columns and is less commonly involved. Many patients are elderly and usually there is little recovery.

SYRINGOMYELIA

This arises from a cystic cavity in the centre of the spinal cord, often in the cervical region. This slowly increases in size acting like an intramedullary spinal tumour (Figure 22).

It is associated with LMN signs in the arms with weak wasted hands, often asymmetrical, and lost arm reflexes. There is usually dissociated sensory loss over the neck, shoulders and arms. Spastic leg weakness is common. Patients often show a kyphoscoliosis.

Patients suspected of a syrinx should be referred to hospital as surgery to the cranio-cervical junction may prevent deterioration.

SUB-ACUTE COMBINED DEGENERATION

This is a combination of a peripheral neuropathy and myelopathy caused by vitamin B12 deficiency. This may also damage the optic nerves and produce a dementia. Although this is associated with pernicious anaemia, patients do not need to be overtly anaemic. B12 deficiency may also arise after gastrectomy, in malabsorption states and in strict vegans.

Patients commonly present with neuropathic symptoms with distal sensory upset – tingling and numbness – associated with limb weakness. The legs feel stiff, weak and unsteady from a combination of spasticity and sensory ataxia (posterior columns). The knee jerks may be brisk, the ankle jerks absent and the plantar responses extensor.

A blood count may show a macrocytic anaemia and the serum B12 level will be low. Referral may be necessary in order to examine the bone marrow and perform a Schilling test on B12 absorption.

Treatment is by large doses by hydroxocobalamin (Neo-Cytamen) by injection 1000 micrograms daily x 10, then once weekly for 6 injections and then once monthly injections for life. Severe or long lasting spinal cord damage may persist.

MOTOR NEURONE DISEASE

This is an uncommon condition causing a progressive loss of motor nerve cells in:

(1)   Anterior horn cells – progressive muscular atrophy.

(2)   The cortico-spinal tract – amyotrophic lateral sclerosis.

(3)   The cranial nerve motor nuclei – progressive bulbar palsy.

Usually all three features are combined although patients may present in different ways. These include:

(1)   A weak wasted hand with LMN signs often spreading to the arm, associated with brisk reflexes, no sensory loss and widespread fasciculation. The distribution initially is often asymmetrical.

(2)   Spastic weakness in one or both legs with a dragging foot, exaggerated reflexes, extensor plantar responses, no sensory loss. Again fasciculations may be visible in the legs, arms and trunk. Sometimes there may be other LMN signs in the legs with wasting. Cramp is a fairly common early symptom.

(3)   About one third present with bulbar weakness leading to complaints about swallowing or speaking. The tongue is weak, wasted and fasciculating. Often there is also an admixture of UMN and LMN signs in the limbs and trunk.

The cause is unknown but there is progressive loss of motor nerve cells. In 10% of patients there is a family history, often showing a dominant inheritance.

Management

The relentless progression usually confirms the diagnosis. Most patients are referred to hospital. It is important to exclude remediable conditions – thyrotoxic myopathy (thyroxine level), polymyositis (CK level), cervical spondylotic radiculomyelopathy (X-rays and myelography), sub-acute combined degeneration (B12 level), a motor neuropathy (EMG studies) and myasthenia gravis (Tensilon test for bulbar symptoms).

Most patients die within three to four years of the diagnosis: those with extensive bulbar symptoms have the worst outlook. There is no specific treatment. Patients and their families will need much support with the provision of disabled aids during this long and harrowing illness. Short duration stays in hospital will give the family a rest.

Symptomatic treatment of cramp with diazepam (Valium), or pains with analgesics, may be necessary. Bulbar weakness leads to swallowing difficulties with 'spill-over' chest infections. Liquidised food and a portable sucker may be some help. Increasing breathlessness, particularly at night, may be managed by sleeping propped up 'sitting' and the use of portable oxygen.

SPINAL CORD COMPRESSION

Presentation

The commonest presenting symptom is *leg weakness*. Mild degrees of weakness may be missed early on and by the time of examination an asymmetrical spastic paraparesis is present. Initially patients may complain of stiffness, heaviness, weakness and fatigue in one or both legs. There may be associated sensory symptoms and signs. Pain and temperature (spinothalamic) sensation are often affected earlier than touch and posterior column modalities. Often the sensory upset appears in the opposite leg to that showing the most spastic weakness (Brown–Séquard's syndrome). Later the sensory loss may become more profound with eventually a clear level on the trunk and involvement of all modalities. The spinal cord ends at the level of L 1 and below that a compressive lesion within the canal will damage the cauda equina.

About one third of patients show an early change in bowel and bladder function. Bladder symptoms include urgency and frequency, later retention with overflow. Increasing constipation may be missed particularly if regular analgesics have been used to counter pain. In the male, impotence may be an early symptom.

Sometimes patients complain of prominent pain either in the back, or in a root distribution at the level of the lesion. Patients may show a scoliosis. Severe back pain while resting in bed always raises the possibility of neoplastic spinal disease. Some patients however, with spinal tumours may have no pain.

Referral

All such patients need early referral for many causes of spinal compression are remediable. Some may need urgent referral for if continued compression occurs it may become critical and 'strangle' the blood supply to the cord causing features similar to a transection. By this time the damage is usually irreversible with total paralysis, complete sensory loss and sphincter failure below the level of the lesion.

Causes

Benign spinal tumours (some 40%) include meningiomata (particularly in middle aged and older women) and neuromata. In older patients often with severe spinal pain, extradural metastatic deposits are common (from cancer of the breast, lung and prostate and also from lymphomas). Abscesses, spinal cord degenerative disorders and disc prolapses (cervical and thoracic) are less common compressive causes.

The family doctor's role

(1) To recognise the early symptoms and signs.
(2) To arrange some investigations in selected patients where the need for referral is not urgent. These include:
   (a) Blood tests – a full blood count, ESR, serum B12, WR or equivalent.
   (b) X-rays of the chest and the appropriate part of the spine. If there is a spastic paraparesis the lesion must be above L 1 so lumbar spine films are not relevant.

FALLS IN THE ELDERLY

Repeated falls in the elderly raises two problems:

(1) Why are they falling?
(2) What can 1 do about it?

Accidents

About one third of such falls are due to accidents. The ageing brain is slow or unable to perceive danger and slower to react to it particularly in terms of reflexes, balance and muscular control. Often vision and hearing may be impaired so afferent input is less acute.

Prevention is better than cure. Attention to lighting, marking steps, handrails, and walking aids are important. It is necessary to stress repeatedly to the elderly the avoidance of going out alone in bad weather, particularly in ice and snow. Discourage climbing on chairs or the use of rickety stepladders. Encourage asking for a helping hand.

Vertebro-basilar ischaemia

This may cause the classic drop attack, most commonly in women. There is sudden falling to the ground with no or only momentary loss of consciousness. It may be associated with vertigo or light-headedness. Less often other symptoms of brain stem ischaemia may occur (page 66). Some attacks may be precipitated by looking up or turning the head suddenly. Minor staggering or giddy sensations without falling are common.

The mechanism is circulatory: some from mechanical interference with hind brain blood flow in the neck, some from fibrin–platelet emboli, and some from changes in cerebral perfusion triggered by blood pressure alterations or disturbances of heart rate or rhythm.

Most patients require reassurance and advice. With a clear history of precipitation by neck movement, a collar may be tried but many elderly patients are very intolerant. Vestibular sedatives are disappointing. Low dose aspirin is sometimes tried.

Syncope (page 37)

The elderly are more prone to fainting and this may be associated with:

(1) Anaemia – take blood for a full count and check for macrocytosis.
(2) Micturition and cough (page 38).
(3) Drugs – particularly hypotensive agents, but also tricyclic anti-depressants, phenothiazines and dopa derivatives. Always ask about any medication.

Parkinson's disease (page 179)

Falls are common. In part this reflects problems with posture, balance and the impairment of righting reflexes. As the disease progresses, falls become more frequent.

Cardiovascular disorders

Changes in heart rate or rhythm, particularly if intermittent, may present with falls and often giddy faint feelings. Some patients also add complaints of palpitations or breathlessness. Persistent pulse irregularities may be detected by examination and a resting ECG. Intermittent faults may require ambulatory ECG monitoring. Some patients may require a pace-maker.

Weakness

This may be spastic or less often flaccid, as discussed previously.

Epilepsy (Chapter 3)

The account of an eye-witness is important, also the duration and circumstances.

Other deficits

In many elderly patients neuronal loss has occurred either from ageing (degeneration) or from the cumulative effects of small strokes (some of these may have been 'silent'). These lead to impaired:

(1) Posture.
(2) Balance.
(3) Righting reflexes.

(4)   Vision and hearing.

(5)   Control of limb co-ordination and strength.

(6)   Mobility with slowing up.

Older patients also show changes in the circulation with inability to adapt to rapid postural change. They also often develop stiff painful 'arthritic' joints.

11

Involuntary Movements

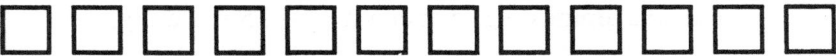

Involuntary movements are a common cause for consultation. Many abnormalities of posture or movement are due to damage in the extrapyramidal pathways – particularly the basal ganglia, and their connexions in the cerebellum and brain stem.

TREMOR

This is a regular alternating rhythmic muscular contraction usually of the distal part of the limbs, but sometimes of the head and trunk. Some tremor is *physiological*. This is fine at about 8 – 12 Hz (previously termed cycles per second) and is made more prominent after exercise. Most pathological tremor is of slower rate.

Parkinsonian

Here tremor is present at rest but decreased by action. The rate is about 3 – 7 Hz and it is aggravated by stress. It often starts in one hand, described as 'pill-rolling'', and may spread into the arm and leg. Later it may involve both sides. It is accompanied by rigidity, cog-wheel in pattern. Blepharoclonus, the fine tremor of lightly closed eye-lids, is part of extrapyramidal tremor. Treatment is described on page 181.

Essential tremor

This is postural, best seen in the out-stretched hands. The rate is about 5 – 8 Hz. It may occur in families with a dominant inheritance, but is also seen sporadically. Commonly the hands are affected but in some 50% the head is involved, and there may be tremor of the jaw, lips and tongue. It is aggravated by stress and often eased by alcohol. Such patients do not show incoordination and walk well.

A number of patients find the tremor helped by propranolol (80 – 120 mg daily), some by primidone (500 – 750 mg daily) and a few by benzodiazepines e.g. diazepam (4 – 15 mg daily).

Intention or ataxic tremor

This is slow, some 2 – 4 Hz and is worse on attempted movement. It is associated with marked incoordination. Such patients commonly show nystagmus, dysarthria and walk unsteadily. A few may show titubation of the head and trunk. Ataxic tremor reflects damage to the cerebellum or its connexions. There are many causes, e.g. MS.

Metabolic disturbances may also cause tremor. These usually produce a fine fast postural tremor. Treatment is of the underlying condition. Causes include: thyrotoxicosis, uraemia and hepatic failure (often a coarse 'flapping' tremor), alcohol, drugs (lithium, caffeine, salbutamol (Ventolin)), anxiety and the "morning shakes" of alcohol withdrawal.

Senile tremor may appear as a combination of rest and action tremor. Some patients show an essential tremor with added extrapyramidal features.

MYOCLONUS

This describes brief shock-like involuntary muscle jerks. These may be single or repeated. They may herald a major epileptic seizure or may arise in rare forms of progressive encephalopathy, e.g. Jakob–Creutzfeldt's disease or Tay–Sachs disease. They can also follow cerebral damage from anoxia, or in uraemia. Some forms of myoclonus may be helped by clonazepam.

TICS AND HABIT SPASMS

These are repetitive stereotyped movements as twitches or facial grimaces commonly seen in the face and hands. There may be utterances or noises. They can be imitated and often appear under stress. A severe form is Gilles de la Tourette syndrome where multiple tics and vocalisations appear – the latter often including obscene words (coprolalia). When severe, tics may respond to haloperidol (0.5 – 5 mg t.i.d.) or pimozide (4 – 10 mg daily).

CHOREA

Here continuous involuntary irregular jerky movements or fidgets occur at random, usually affecting the face and limbs. They are not stereotyped and are not predictable. Such patients have difficulty holding their arms out-stretched and if they are then held above the head, they may hyperpronate. Testing grip shows this to be irregular and tongue protrusion may prove difficult. The gait is often odd, 'dancing', with at times 'piano-playing' fidgets in the fingers.

Chorea may arise as:

Sydenham's (St. Vitus' Dance)

About one third show rheumatic cardiac involvement. This is now rarely seen, usually in children.

Chorea gravidarum

This appears in pregnancy or with the contraceptive pill (OC pill).

Drugs

For example, phenytoin, lithium, 'dopa' preparations, OC pill.

Medical

Polycythaemia rubra vera, thyrotoxicosis, systemic lupus erythematosus.

Huntington's

This is a *dominant inherited degenerative disease* affecting the caudate nuclei and the frontal and temporal lobes. It causes chorea and a progressive dementia. Patients may present with involuntary movements but more often with changes of personality, behaviour and failing memory which may be more apparent to others. Most patients present in middle age but may survive some 15 years or more. Most end in psychiatric hospitals.

Thiopropazate (5 – 10 mg t.i.d.), haloperidol (0.5 – 5 mg t.i.d.) or tetrabenazine (25 mg t.i.d.) may reduce the choreic fidgets. Genetic advice is often sought. There is a 50:50 chance of any child of an affected patient developing the disease.

A more dramatic *hemichorea* involving proximal limb muscles on one side so the limbs are forcefully flung about is termed *hemiballismus*. This is most often seen after a stroke in the opposite sub-thalamic nucleus. A phenothiazine as chlorpromazine (25 mg t.i.d.) or drug as tetrabenazine (25 mg t.i.d.) may reduce the movements although these often settle spontaneously given time.

ATHETOSIS

This describes continuous writhing involuntary movements with the inability to maintain the limbs in one posture. Often such movements are combined with choreic fidgets. These are most commonly seen with childhood brain damage.

DYSTONIA

Here there is spasm of the limbs, head or trunk, usually persisting in some unusual position. Rare diseases as dystonia musculorum deformans, or Wilson's disease may present in this way. More common are drug-induced acute dystonias, most often seen in young women and provoked by:

(1)   phenothiazines, e.g. prochlorperazine, perphenazine

(2)   metoclopramide.

More *chronic dystonic postures* may also arise from long term use of *phenothiazines, butyrophenones* or *thioxanthenes*. These dystonias may be associated with choreic fidgets and sometimes signs of Parkinsonism with an immobile face, marked rigidity and slowness. These may take many weeks to improve after the drugs have been stopped particularly if depot injections have been used, e.g. fluphenazine (Modecate).

Another group of more serious drug-induced involuntary movements are the *tardive dyskinesias* where oro-facial movements are prominent with often distal chorea and trunk rocking. Such movements may appear some six months or more after continuous treatment with phenothiazines or haloperidol and a significant number do not reverse when the drugs are stopped.

FOCAL DYSTONIAS

These may occur in a number of conditions:

Spasmodic torticollis 'wry neck'

Here there is sustained spasm of the sternomastoid on one side causing the head to turn. In chronic instances the affected muscles may hypertrophy.

Writer's cramp

This is a specific inability to write. The fingers holding the pen seem to go into spasm with an odd posture. Other fine manipulative tasks, such as using tools, are unaffected.

Blepharospasm, oro-mandibular dystonia, Breughel's syndrome

Older patients may show spasm of the orbicularis oculi with eye closure severe enough to render them partially sighted. The facial muscles and speech may also be disturbed.

Treatment

In all focal dystonias drug therapy is disappointing but a trial of benzhexol (2 – 10 mg daily) and diazepam (2 – 5 mg t.i.d.) is worthwhile. Some patients are treated surgically.

HEMIFACIAL SPASM

This affects middle aged and older patients, women more than men. Fine repetitive twitching appears in one cheek often making the eye wink. This may spread into the whole face on one side causing some asymmetry. The cause is usually unknown but rarely it may follow a Bell's palsy or facial nerve irritation from a cerebellopontine angle tumour. It is important to differentiate from *myokymia*, a continuous fine rippling in the cheek muscles, most often seen in brain stem lesions as MS.

Hemifacial spasm responds poorly to drugs but diazepam, clonazepam and carbamazepine are worth a trial. In a few patients posterior fossa exploration has shown an arterial branch in contact with the facial nerve. If this is moved away from the nerve this will give relief.

RESTLESS LEGS (EKBOM'S SYNDROME)

Patients complain of aching and discomfort in the feet and legs at rest and particularly in bed at night. This discomfort is so intense that they often get up and walk about. A few have cramps as well and dislike the weight of the bed clothes. The cause is unknown; in a few iron deficiency anaemia or uraemia has been found. Many respond to clonazepam 0.5 − 1 mg nocte.

12

Multiple Sclerosis

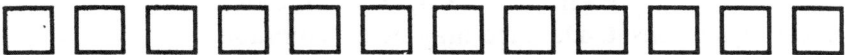

Multiple sclerosis (MS) causes multiple patches (plaques) of demyelination affecting the white matter of the CNS with anatomical and temporal dissemination. The *aetiology* is still unknown although GPs will be asked about current theories. One is that the cause is a 'slow virus' to which the patient is exposed in the first five to fifteen years of life. This then provokes an inflammatory disturbance in susceptible patients who turn their defences (auto-immunity) against their own CNS myelin. At present, despite claims, there is no clear single diagnostic test which confirms the disease although a number may support the diagnosis.

INCIDENCE

The prevalence in the UK is approximately 1:2000 and young adults are most often affected, women more than men (3:2). The peak age of incidence is about 30 years. In older patients, particularly middle aged males, the disease may present with a slowly progressive spastic paraperesis. However, patients usually show relapses and remissions. After the latter there may be worsening recovery with resulting cumulative disability. The mean duration of the disease is about twenty years.

171

The GP is faced with two groups:

(1) *New patients* – here the question is one of diagnosis – is this MS?

(2) *Old patients* with known MS. These may have fresh neurological upset, or persistent problems from chronic or progressive disability.

DIAGNOSIS IN NEW PATIENTS

Patients may present with single or multiple symptoms of neurological upset. Damage may occur commonly in:

(1) The *optic nerves* with sudden *visual loss* or blurring, an optic neuritis (page 88).

(2) The *spinal cord*, often in the cervical region. Posterior column sensory loss may lead to complaints of a *useless hand*, numbness or tingling, or even electric shock sensations provoked by neck flexion (Lhermitte's phenomenon). Corticospinal tract involvement will cause weakness, heaviness and stiffness of a *leg* with *spastic weakness*. Although the complaint is of a fault in one leg, often there are signs in both. There may be signs of posterior column sensory upset in both feet. Intermedio-lateral column involvement will cause micturition upset – *urgency* and *frequency*, later retention with overflow, constipation, and in the male, *impotence* (Figure 22).

(3) The *brain stem* with balance upset, visual symptoms and often involvement of the long tracts passing through to the limbs. Cerebellar disturbance leads to incoordination in the limbs, an intention tremor, scanning dysarthria, *ataxy* of *stance* and *gait* and often nystagmus (page 66). *Double vision* may arise from an internuclear ophthalmoplegia (page 101) or an abducens or oculomotor palsy. There may be *facial sensory* upset, *trigeminal neuralgia*, myokymia, or even an LMN *facial palsy*. Episodes of acute *vertigo* with prostration may also occur (page 64).

With prolonged disease many patients may show a degree of *dementia*. There is often *depression* and *euphoria*, perhaps from frontal plaques.

Past episodes

In new patients it is always worth inquiring about any past neurological symptoms.

Signs

The presence of signs often indicates the need for hospital referral although in mild attacks this may not be necessary. At hospital investigations may include evoked potential studies (visual, auditory or somato-sensory) and often a CSF examination (some 75% of MS patients show an elevated IgG value in the CSF protein and some 90% may show the presence of oligoclonal bands on protein electrophoresis).

Treatment

Many patients make spontaneous full recoveries from early episodes. In *acute relapses* rest and a short course of *steroids* may speed recovery, although they do not influence the degree of that recovery. ACTH injections are often used – in doses of 80 units, 60 units and 40 units, for five days at each dose. Steroids should not be given in prolonged courses as they have no value and produce unwanted side effects.

Symptomatic treatment may also be helpful, as anti-emetics for acute vomiting, or carbamazepine for neuralgia or transient paroxysmal disorders. Physiotherapy helps patients with limb and gait problems.

Diet

Many have been claimed to be beneficial – these include added vitamins, vitamin B12 injections, the addition of polyunsaturated fatty acids (sunflower seed oil), a fat-free diet and a gluten-free diet. Although these have their supporters, the authors are not convinced of their efficacy and this is supported by statistics. The most hopeful studies have come from the use of polyunsaturated fatty acids.

Trials

Other trials are currently in progress using immuno-suppressants (the MRC Azathioprine trial) and the use of hyperbaric oxygen in a decompression chamber. The results are not available yet.

When to tell the patient?

There is debate about this but the authors believe it is not advisable to tell patients after a single episode. The diagnosis may be wrong and such patients may have no further attacks. However, if a patient has repeated episodes, and investigations support the diagnosis of MS and have excluded a number of other possibilities (e.g. a spinal tumour), then it is important to discuss the diagnosis with the patient and their relatives.

THE CHRONIC PATIENT

Deterioration may follow an acute relapse. Sometimes this may be from a further attack, or from an intercurrent infection or even some other insult, e.g. trauma or surgery. Correction of any infection is important, e.g. urinary tract.

Such patients may require admission particularly if:

(1) The acute relapse causes uncontrolled symptoms, e.g. vomiting, vertigo, bulbar weakness or severe limb weakness.

(2) The home facilities are such that they cannot be nursed at home. A small number of young chronic sick in institutions are MS patients.

(3) To give relatives a rest or holiday.

Relapses follow the pattern of the acute episodes but the chronic patient may also have:

Sphincter problems

Constipation

Bowel opening with an appropriate diet may be sufficient to establish a fairly regular action. Bulk preparations as bran and sterculia (Normacol) may help some patients. In more refractory problems, suppositories – glycerine, and bisacodyl (Dulcolax), may act as a stimulant, but if these fail then an enema or manual removal may sometimes prove necessary.

Bladder problems

Urgency and frequency of micturition may have a neurogenic basis but it is essential to check that there is no infection (urine culture). Fluid restriction in the late evening together with drugs as propantheline (Pro-Banthine) or emepronium (Cetiprin), with a loading dose given at bed-time may aid some patients.

Incontinence is a major handicap. In the male a number of penile appliances may prove effective providing there is a good fit for the sheath to prevent leakage, particularly while the patient is lying. In the female appliances are far less satisfactory. Measures include incontinence pads, intermittent self-catheterisation, and an indwelling catheter. The last of course is necessary if there is significant retention. Long term catheters create their own problems with infections and their retrograde spread to the kidneys. A few patients have found benefit from major surgery with a urinary diversion to an ileal conduit. Such patients will be referred to urologists with a special interest in these difficulties.

Spasticity

In patients with spastic leg weakness, this will make walking more difficult as the legs stiffen, the thighs tend to adduct and the feet plantarflex. Reduction of this may aid walking but it is important not to reduce this too far and replace the stiffness by flaccid weakness, so that the legs buckle under the patient's weight. Paraplegic patients with little movement in the legs may have distressing flexor spasms, and the legs may be drawn up rigid in flexion, or sometimes extended in a painful position. Such postures may interfere with patients obtaining a comfortable sitting position.

A number of drugs may reduce spasticity but these all have side effects.

(1) Baclofen (Lioresal) 15 – 60 mg daily in divided doses is the authors' first preference. The dose needs to be gradually increased. In high doses it may cause confusion, provoke epileptic seizures or hypotension.

(2) Diazepam (Valium) given in doses of 15 – 40 mg daily. Unfortunately this often causes sedation but a bed-time dose may be helpful.

(3) Dantrolene sodium (Dantrium) 25 – 300 mg daily given in divided doses. Again the dose should be increased slowly. It may cause drowsiness, dizziness and rarely liver upset so liver function tests are advised while using this.

Very severe flexor spasms, doubling a patient up, may require destruction of neural pathways. Such patients may be referred to hospital with a view to a phenol 'block' of appropriate lumbar or sacral roots. Such measures may disturb bowel and bladder function.

176

Care of the skin

Immobility with incontinence often result in pressure sores developing in paralysed patients. This is more likely if there is also sensory loss in the affected area. Such patients may then develop horrifying deep ulcers even eroding underlying bone and producing a low grade osteomyelitis. Often there is secondary anaerobic infection in such lesions. These ulcers may lead to systemic upset and anaemia.

The most important aspect is prevention with regular turning of patients at risk. Large ulcers may need admission to hospital with a view to skin grafting and surgical cleansing. Anaemia may require transfusion. Small ulcers may be managed at home often with the help of the community nurse for regular dressings.

Provision of aids

A home assessment visit by the community occupational therapist will give help in determining a number of aids for daily living. These include extra rails in the bathroom, around the lavatory, and on the stairs. Also advice can be obtained with regard to more major additions or alterations such as the installation of a lift, provision of a shower with a ramp for the shower chair, and even an electric hoist. Families may get some financial help for these from local authorities.

Walking aids may best be provided with the help of a physiotherapist. More disabled patients may need the provision of a wheelchair – the most commonly used being the lightweight folding pattern with large outer wheels which patients can turn with their hands.

Courses of physiotherapy, and hydrotherapy, may prove very helpful.

MS society

This is a far reaching organisation with many active local branches. It provides information, social activities and gives help and support for members and their families, e.g. in provision of holiday facilities. It collects funds and finances research into the disease.

Chronic MS patients or their families may ask about:

(1) *Inheritance* There appears to be an increased risk of developing MS in first degree relatives, probably highest in sibs. The use of HLA tissue typing has shown that there seems an increase of HLA3 in such patients.

(2) *Pregnancy* There is no particular increased risk of relapse during pregnancy although there does seem to be a slightly increased risk in the first few months post-partum; perhaps tied in with the increased work load. Parents with MS should be advised not to have large families.

(3) *Risks of relapse* These appear more common if patients become very over-tired, after viral infections particularly with a high temperature, and rarely after some immunisations.

(4) *Fatigue* This is a troublesome symptom and proves difficult to treat. In a small number of patients this is so marked that they lead the life of an invalid, may appear very depressed, and may need psychiatric treatment. Patients with physical disability will tire more easily. There is a physiological basis for this in that nerve fibres with an inadequate myelin sheath, may actually develop a transient conduction block if the temperature is raised, or fail to conduct repeated trains of impulses. This may explain why many patients are aware that their symptoms are worse when fatigued or if they become hot.

13

Parkinson's Disease

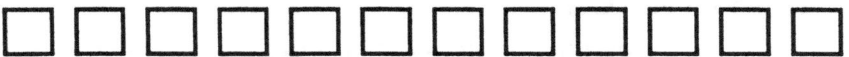

The diagnosis of Parkinson's disease (Shaking Palsy) is clinical and rests on:

(1) *Rigidity*, of cog-wheel type.

(2) *Slowness of movement*, bradykinesia or hypokinesia.

(3) *Tremor*, at 3 – 7 Hz. This is worst at rest, often disappearing as a movement is started. It is often described as 'pill-rolling' in the hand.

CLINICAL

Patients may present with an insidious onset of weakness or inability to use a hand for fine manipulative tasks and this slowly worsens. Writing deteriorates becoming smaller – micrographia. Tremor may be present at the onset in two thirds of patients. In walking there may be dragging of one foot with poverty of arm swing. Symptoms often start on one side, later they may become bilateral. Balance and posture are affected with problems in turning or walking through a narrow space. There is difficulty getting out of a low chair or the bath. Speech may become soft and fade. There may be excessive salivation with distressing dribbling.

Later patients complain of frequent falls and that their feet 'freeze' as though stuck to the ground. The gait may become festinant, tending to break into a run and this is associated with a flexed posture. Patients walk with short shuffling paces.

Repetitive movements are poorly performed and the face appears immobile – impassive. Constipation may develop. Many patients become depressed. In the later stages some patients become demented. A few patients may develop autonomic disturbances with postural hypotension, sweating crises and urinary incontinence.

PATHOPHYSIOLOGY

In most patients Parkinson's disease is due to a neuronal degeneration of unknown cause which affects the nigro-striatal pathways in the basal ganglia. Despite treatment the nerve cell loss progresses accounting for the deterioration. In a few patients symptoms may follow repeated trauma (punch-drunk boxers), carbon monoxide poisoning, encephalitis or more often the use of phenothiazines or butyrophenones. Parkinsonian symptoms may also appear as part of a more widespread neuronal degeneration as in progressive supra-nuclear palsy (page 100), or multi-system atrophy.

NEUROTRANSMITTERS

A number of neurotransmitters are recognised. Dopamine, an inhibitory transmitter, normally is concentrated in the basal ganglia. In Parkinson's disease it is depleted. One of its antagonistic excitatory transmitters is acetylcholine. Treatment of Parkinson's disease relies on trying to increase the brain dopamine or decrease the acetylcholine. Phenothiazines and butyrophenones block dopamine receptors.

INCIDENCE AND NATURAL HISTORY

This increases in the elderly with a value of one in 100 – 200 over the age of sixty, and a mean age of onset of fifty-five. Prior to the use of 'dopa' preparations most patients died within ten years of onset but it appears that 'dopa' treatment prolongs life expectancy. Some two thirds of patients respond to 'dopa' but about one third do not. Of the responders with more prolonged use, nearly two thirds find loss of benefit over the next three to five years. Patients who deteriorate are often elderly with increasing disability, immobility and frequent falls. In some they become bed-ridden, helpless and even may develop a terminal bronchopneumonia. Others may fall fracturing a hip and the further immobility leads to greater restriction of activity. Any intercurrent illness may cause a temporary deterioration.

TREATMENT

Mildly affected patients should try:

Anti-cholinergic drugs, e.g.

Benzhexol (Artane) 4 – 15 mg daily in divided doses.

Orphenadrine (Disipal) 150 – 300 mg daily in divided doses.

Benztropine (Cogentin) 2 – 6 mg daily given at bed-time.

Side effects:

These may all cause parasympathetic blockade with a dry mouth, constipation, blurred vision, a tendency to urinary retention and *confusion* (particularly in the elderly).

Amantadine (Symmetrel) 100 – 200 mg daily given in the morning and at noon to avoid insomnia.

Side effects:

This may produce oedema, skin changes (livedo reticularis) and occasionally confusion.

Amantadine and anti-cholinergic drugs are synergistic and they can all be combined and also used together with 'dopa' preparations.

More severely affected patients should try:

Levodopa (L 3,4 dihydroxyphenylalanine) – 'dopa'. This is the precursor of dopamine and is converted to this by the action of dopa decarboxylase (DDC). If 'dopa' is given by mouth most of it is converted by DDC in the gut and tissues into dopamine which cannot cross the blood–brain barrier and so is not available in the brain. 'Dopa', however, can cross the blood–brain barrier. By combining 'dopa' with a DDC inhibitor (the inhibitor does not cross the barrier) a small dose of 'dopa' can be used which enters the brain. Here it is converted into dopamine by the brain DDC.

Combined preparations include:

(1)   Dopa and carbidopa – Sinemet.

(2)   Dopa and benserazide – Madopar.

Either of these combined preparations may be introduced in a low dose (Madopar – 125 or Sinemet – 110), e.g. one tablet or capsule b.d. p.c. and this dose is then slowly increased to produce benefit. A stronger preparation is also available, Madopar – 250 which contains 200 mg of 'dopa', and Sinemet – 275 which contains 250 mg of 'dopa'. In the very elderly a lower dose may be necessary on starting treatment, e.g. Madopar – 62.5 (which contains 50 mg of 'dopa') or a half tablet of Sinemet – 110 (also contains 50 mg of 'dopa'), as such patients seem much more sensitive.

Side effects:

These include nausea and vomiting, dyskinetic involuntary movements (particularly dose-related), postural hypotension, confusion and even psychosis.

About two thirds of patients respond to 'dopa' in combined form but after three to five years these benefits may lessen. The deterioration may follow:

(1)   Return of increasingly severe Parkinsonian symptoms, particularly immobility and postural upset. Some of these patients also appear demented. Often the response to further treatment is disappointing but benefit from smaller 'dopa' doses given more frequently may occur.

(2) Fluctuations in performance with periods of relatively good mobility alternating with periods of marked immobility – the *'on–off' phenomenon*. Such patients may show end-dose deterioration suggesting they may need more frequent doses of 'dopa' but they may also show an increase in dyskinesia about 40 – 60 minutes after their last 'dopa' dose, peak-dose dyskinesia. Some patients show increased tremor in their 'off' periods. These swings may be severe causing marked immobility, frequent falls and increasing disability. It is worth trying as treament:

(a) Smaller doses of 'dopa' given more often, e.g. two hourly.

(b) The addition of a dopamine-agonist as *bromocriptine (Parlodel)*. Usually the starting dose is 2.5 mg daily and this is increased slowly to 20 – 40 mg daily. The 'dopa' dose may need to be reduced. Side effects are similar to those found with 'dopa' but psychiatric disturbances are more common, occur at a lower dose and may persist longer.

(c) The addition of *selegiline (Eldepryl)*, a selective monoamine oxidase B inhibitor, starting with 5 mg mane and increasing to 5 mg mane and noon. Again the 'dopa' dose may need to be reduced. Only about half the patients with 'on–off' symptoms respond to this. Side effects include hypotension, nausea, vomiting and confusion.

DEPRESSION

This is a common problem and responds to conventional treatment. Tricyclic anti-depressants given as a single dose at bed–time may be effective, e.g. amitriptyline (Tryptizol) 50 – 75 mg nocte. Nomifensine (Merital) 25 – 50 mg b.d. to t.i.d. may also be useful as it has some dopamine-agonist activity.

Physiotherapy is helpful. If mobility is maintained patients seem

183

to 'seize up' less and problems such as 'freezing' or walking through narrow spaces may be overcome. Assessment at home by an occupational therapist with a view to the provision of various aids in the bathroom, for dressing, and to check that beds and chairs are at an appropriate level for the patient, is worthwhile.

There is a *Parkinson's Disease Society* where patients and their relatives may receive helpful advice and support.

Always check patients with Parkinson's disease to see that:

(1)   They are not hypothyroid.

(2)   They are not depressed.

(3)   They are not on any drugs which cause or aggravate the condition.

FAILURE OF TREATMENT

If patients with 'Parkinsonism' fail to respond well to treatment always consider, is this a more widespread neuronal degeneration (Parkinsonism-Plus)? Such patients need specialist referral.

14
The Unconscious Patient, Head Injuries

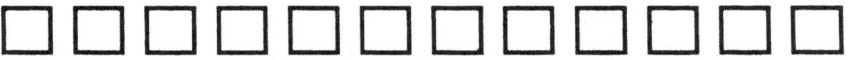

THE UNCONSCIOUS PATIENT

The common presentation is as an emergency, often in an atmosphere of panic: the patient is unconscious and cannot be roused.

On the telephone

Ensure that details of the name and address are obtained, and if available, the patient's age. Are there signs of major injuries (bleeding, or obvious broken limbs) as these might make the ordering of an ambulance at this stage helpful? Advise the caller to check the patient is lying on their side with a free airway.

Before leaving

Obtain any available records.

On arrival

(1) Check the airway. Are there any signs of respiratory upset,

cyanosis or obstruction? Are there signs of shock? Deal with any life-threatening complications, e.g. airway obstruction, arterial bleeding.

(2) Determine briefly the level of consciousness – any verbal response, state of eyes, limb movements to pain (Table 12). Note the time.

(3) If necessary summon an ambulance to arrange transfer to hospital.

Now there is time to hear from:

(a) Relatives or bystanders with regard to the circumstances.

(b) Check any past medical history of relevance – particularly diabetes, heart trouble.

(c) Find out if they are on any current drugs. Check the surrounds for tablet bottles, alcohol, syringes, medical cards or suicide notes.

Table 12 Assessment of conscious level

Best verbal response	Orientated
	Confused
	Inappropriate
	Incomprehensible
	None
Best motor response	Obeying
	Localising
	Flexing ⎫
	Extending ⎬ to pain
	None ⎭
Eye opening response	Spontaneous
	To speech
	To pain
	None

After Teasdale and Jennett (1974)[26]

Re-assess the patient with a more detailed examination

Often the patient recovers consciousness after a fairly brief interval. Note are they confused? Can they give an account of what has happened? Do they have a severe headache?

Check the *level of consciousness again* if they have not recovered.

Check the *pupils* (page 10). Do they react? Are the *eyes* still or roving?

Are they deviated to one side as may follow frontal brain damage (page 99)?

If the head is turned from side to side, will the eyes turn to the opposite side – *doll's head eye movements*? If they do, this indicates the brain stem pathway is intact. Check the *fundi*. Are there signs of disc swelling or haemorrhages?

Check the *respiratory rate and rhythm*. A waxing and waning pattern, Cheyne–Stokes breathing may be present. This is most often seen in bihemisphere damage but can also occur with metabolic upsets. If respiration is disturbed again make certain there is no airway obstruction. Check if there is a smell of ketones or alcohol on the breath, but remember that the smell of alcohol does not exclude other serious conditions as head injury or stroke. Blood alcohol levels of 300 – 400 mg/100 ml are necessary to render a patient comatose.

Check if there is a *'gag' reflex*.

Check the *pulse rate and rhythm*, and the *blood pressure*. Is the patient shocked?

Check for signs of *injury*. Are there signs of bruising of the head or face, bleeding from the nose, ears or mouth, extensive trunk bruising, or abnormal postures in the limbs or neck?

Check is the patient *febrile*? Do they have signs of *meningism?*

Check the *limbs* for any evidence of focal deficit. If there is a depressed conscious level, do the limbs respond equally by withdrawal to a painful stimulus? A flaccid weakness on one side may suggest a hemiparesis. Reflex asymmetries and extensor plantar responses may help.

187

Check have they been *incontinent* of urine or faeces, or have they *vomited*?
Check is there any evidence of *systemic upset* – jaundice, skin rashes, abdominal distension?

The common causes of loss of consciousness include:

Syncope – faints
Epilepsy
      Febrile convulsions in children
Breath-holding attacks in children
Self-poisoning   drugs and alcohol
Metabolic upset
      Diabetes mellitus   diabetic coma (slower onset)
                                hypoglycaemia

      Uraemia
      Hepatic failure
      B1 deficiency   Wernicke's encephalopathy
Trauma
Vascular disease
      Cerebral haemorrhage   Sub-arachnoid haemorrhage
                             Haemorrhagic infarction
      Thrombo-embolic infarction
Infections
      Meningitis   bacterial, viral
      Encephalitis   herpes simplex
      Cerebral abscess
      Septicaemia
      Cerebral malaria

Cerebral tumours
    Mass effect   primary or metastatic
    Obstructive hydrocephalus
    Raised intracranial pressure
Anoxia
    Cardio-respiratory failure
    Myocardial infarction
Hysteria

Management

This depends on the diagnosis and whether the unconscious state persists. Unless there is rapid spontaneous recovery most patients will be transferred to hospital by ambulance. Hypoglycaemic 'coma' will respond to 20 – 30 ml of 50% glucose given intravenously.

An epileptic seizure in a known epileptic patient may only require a check that no serious injury has occurred and that there has been good drug compliance. If the last is in doubt a blood sample taken at this time will allow the levels to be measured to see if adjustments in the dose are necessary. A first epileptic seizure requires further assessment, often referral to hospital for an outpatient appointment. Status epilepticus is a medical emergency requiring urgent control of seizures and admission (page 54). Febrile convulsions in children require admission usually and are discussed on page 55.

Patients remaining unconscious after an epileptic or apoplectic seizure may have also sustained a head injury. Elderly patients may have had a stroke. All patients with significant depression of conscious level from drugs or alcohol, particularly if there are any signs of injury, require admission.

A high temperature or meningism suggests an infective process. Such patients need urgent admission as delay adversely affects the outcome. Meningism may also follow intracranial bleeding.

The presence of fixed dilated pupils, absent brain stem reflexes (gag, corneal, doll's head eye movements) and absent limb responses to pain or decerebrate posturing (limbs extending) are bad prognostic features. If these signs, however, are due to drugs, some patients may recover.

HEAD INJURIES

These are very common. Over 100,000 patients are admitted to hospital in the UK each year with a head injury, but only some 5% of these are admitted or transferred to a neurosurgical unit.

The severity of a closed head injury may in part be assessed by the duration of *post-traumatic amnesia* (PTA). PTA is the duration of loss of memory from the time of injury to recovery of continuous recall of ongoing events. A PTA of more than 24 hours duration indicates a severe head injury. Patients with penetrating head injuries may not lose consciousness.

Patients who are seen while they are still unconscious need hospital admission. It is important to *secure their airway* and position them in a semi-prone position for the journey. Other injuries may need attention. A very brief examination will show if the pupils react and are equal and whether there is any focal deficit. Such details should be noted together with the time and sent with the patient to hospital.

The majority of head injuries are mild and there may have been only brief loss of consciousness or amnesia. Many such patients are conscious or recovering consciousness at the time they are seen.

Hospital referral

Patients should be referred to hospital if there is any evidence of:

(1) Altered conscious level or confusion. Children particularly may appear drowsy, seem muddled and may vomit.

(2) Abnormal neurological signs, e.g. weakness, pupillary inequality.

(3) Bleeding or fluid discharge from the ears or nose.

(4) Suspicion of a penetrating head injury.

(5) A skull fracture – this may be depressed.

(6) A severe scalp laceration.

(7) Fractures of the face, jaw or nose.

(8) An eye injury.

(9) Epileptic seizures.

(10) Suspicion of alcohol or drug ingestion plus head injury.

(11) Prolonged duration of loss of consciousness (5 – 10 minutes or more), or amnesia of more than a few minutes.

(12) Severe headache with vomiting, or any suggestion of meningism.

What is controversial is whether brief loss of consciousness, of about five minutes duration, needs referral. In many instances such patients can be managed at home providing there is a responsible relative who can continue observation with instructions to report any deterioration of conscious level or untoward developments.

Extradural haematoma

The fear after a head injury is the development of an extra-cerebral collection of blood which then causes acute brain compression. This may arise from arterial bleeding, often from a torn middle meningeal artery, or less often from an acute subdural haematoma. Commonly these are associated with parietal or temporal skull fractures although children may show no skull fracture. Such extradural bleeding is uncommon, about 36 per million population each year. However, early recognition of such patients at risk is essential as with delay the outcome may prove fatal.

Such bleeding usually develops within 24 – 36 hours after the injury. Most patients show a progressive deterioration of consciousness although many give the classical history of a head injury with altered consciousness, followed by a relatively lucid interval, and then progressive deterioration. In adults who are *confused or disorientated* after a head injury, and show evidence of a *skull fracture*, one in four will develop an intracranial haematoma[27].

Important symptoms are:

(1) Confusion or disorientation.

(2) Increasing drowsiness with a deteriorating conscious level.

(3) Increasing headache and vomiting.

(4) The development of focal signs, sometimes these are bilateral, e.g. extensor plantar responses.

(5) Abnormal pupillary responses – an enlarging unreactive pupil, also lost upgaze.

(6) A falling pulse with rising blood pressure or altered respiration.

In patients who are already unconscious it is further deterioration with the appearance of focal features and pupillary changes which are important. Venous bleeding causing subdural haematomata may have a slower evolution (page 32).

Patients observed at home

A doctor leaving a patient in the hands of a reliable observer must give clear instructions as what to look for, and the indications for summoning assistance. Advice will also be necessary about the best simple analgesics to use for headaches, and if recovery is proceeding uneventfully, guidelines about diet and mobilisation. Later advice will be necessary about when to return to work or school.

Residual sequelae

After major head injury some patients are left with significant *physical* and/or *mental disability*, some 1,500 such patients in the UK each year. Physical handicap may be so severe as to leave a patient totally dependent, confined to bed or a wheelchair. Various deficits may persist; spastic weakness, tremor, extrapyramidal signs, unsteadiness, disturbed speech, impaired vision or hearing, or loss of other senses.

Brain damage may also cause significant changes in intellectual function with memory impairment, learning failure, altered behaviour and personality. Sometimes these changes are much more of a handicap to a patient returning to work or taking their place in the family. Discussion with relatives will often elicit valuable details about such changes.

There is considerable potential for the recovery of physical deficits particularly in younger patients. Most recovery occurs within the first six months. Older patients, aged more than 50, adapt far less well to significant head injuries. As a rough guideline to the time a patient may take to return to work, most patients with a PTA of one hour or less will be back at work within eight weeks, but if the PTA was 24 hours or more than it may be 4 – 6 months before they return. Obviously with very mild injuries the duration is very much shorter. The severely disabled may need residential care. Attendance at day centres may ease pressure on the family. Active rehabilitation programmes may be available and prove very valuable.

Post-traumatic epilepsy

About 5% of patients with closed head injuries and about 50% of those with penetrating injuries have continuing epileptic seizures. Within four years of the injury some 80% of patients who are going to develop post-traumatic epilepsy will have had a seizure.

About 5% of patients admitted to hospital with head injuries have a fit in the first week. The risks of developing post-traumatic epilepsy later on have shown to be significantly increased by certain factors – an acute intracranial haematoma (31%), early epilepsy in the first week (25%), and a depressed skull fracture (15%). If none of these factors are present then the risks in a closed head injury are only about 1%[28].

Post-traumatic syndrome – post-concussive states

After a head injury with often only brief loss of consciousness or little or no amnesia, some patients complain bitterly of headache (page 31), dizziness, faint feelings, blurred vision, poor concentration and memory. These symptoms may be accompanied by irritability, insomnia, depression and loss of libido. Patients often complain their symptoms are worsened by physical or mental effort and by noise.

Such symptoms may settle within a few weeks but in a proportion of patients, often after very minor injuries, may persist for a surprisingly long time. They are often aggravated if there is a compensation issue at stake. These have been labelled as 'accident neurosis' by Miller[29]. Patients with severe head injuries and children rarely develop post-concussive symptoms.

Often rest, reassurance and regular simple analgesics with sometimes an anti-depressant may prove helpful. Many patients require hospital referral if the symptoms persist.

Head injury prevention

Family doctors may be asked to talk to schools, community groups or advise patients about potential head and spinal injury risks. These particularly include:

(1)   Vehicles. Motor vehicles cause some 60% of head injuries. Motor cyclists have a very high risk of head, spinal and brachial plexus injuries, despite the use of a protective helmet.

(2)   Roads. The very old and very young show a high accident risk.

(3)   Sports. Rugby, boxing, diving, horse riding and the use of trampolines carry a high risk.

(4)   Work. In certain occupations, e.g. miners, scaffolders, protective helmets should be worn.

15

Spinal Cord Injuries

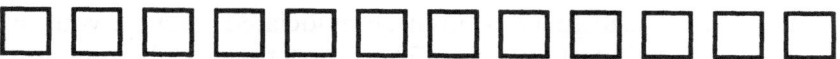

Guttmann[30] with his unique experience of some 2,000 patients treated at the Spinal Injuries Unit at Stoke Mandeville Hospital found some 898 complete, 604 incomplete and 461 cauda equina lesions. The incidence of injuries at different levels was:

Cervical	24%
Upper thoracic	10%
Lower thoracic	43%
Cauda equina	23%
Cervical	15%
Upper thoracic	16%
Lower thoracic	69%

The lumbar segments of the spinal cord lie opposite T 10 – 12 vertebrae. Below the level of L 2 damage involves the cauda equina.

CORD DAMAGE

This may result from direct injuries – missile injuries or stab wounds: these are rare except in wartime. It may also follow indirect injuries – most often car accidents, sporting injuries (diving, rugby) or in falls downstairs, particularly if drunk. The commonest level affected is in the lower thoracic region where a complete lesion will paralyse the legs and cause loss of bowel and

195

bladder control. Neck injuries may follow acute flexion from a relatively mild insult. The most commonly affected level is at C 5/6. If the lesion is at C 3/4 or above, the diaphragm may be paralysed and patients will require ventilation for survival. If there is paralysis of the legs and hands, this suggests a lesion at C 6/7 or above. If the arms can only be abducted and flexed at the shoulders, the lesion is likely to be at C 5/6.

SPINAL DAMAGE

With cord damage there is often an associated fracture with or without dislocation of the spine. The dislocation may be transient and sometimes may spontaneously reduce. In children the spinal cord may be damaged without evidence of a fracture.

GPs are likely to be called to the roadside or sports field. Patients may also have an associated head injury with loss of consciousness. Often there is a vertebral injury.

If conscious, pain may be felt at the site of injury or in the corresponding segmental distribution. Such pain may arise from damaged nerve roots or bone or soft tissue damage. Patients may complain that they cannot move or feel their legs.

EXAMINATION

Shortly after injury check:

(1) That respiration is satisfactory. A high cervical cord lesion may cause respiratory failure.

(2) Is the patient shocked?

(3) Is there tenderness at the site of the lesion?

(4) Is there weakness or paralysis of the limbs? At this stage the legs may appear flaccid with lost reflexes.

(5) Is there sensory loss below a particular level? Marked sensory loss in the hands suggests damage above C 5.

FIRST AID

A high index of suspicion and care in moving the patient is important to prevent further damage if there is an unstable spinal fracture. In some patients cord damage worsens after the accident. J. Brice suggested at his lecture on Spinal Cord Injuries given at Ashford Post-Graduate Medical Centre in 1984, that the early deterioration in a spinal cord injury may be due to the development of haemorrhagic lesions in the watershed territory in the cord between the distribution of the anterior and posterior spinal arteries. To overcome this it may be worth in the first few hours adding oxygen (by mask), a plasma expander and even a dopamine infusion.

At the scene:

(1) Secure the airway and check there is adequate ventilatory function.

(2) Briefly check movement and sensation in the limbs.

(3) Obtain trained help to move the patient. It is likely to be ambulance men. Prevent well-wishers from moving the patient.

(4) In moving patients with suspected spinal damage the principle is to avoid any undue flexion or extension of the spine, particularly the neck. Sufficient helpers are important – ideally at least four. One to apply gentle traction to the head and support it, a second to manage the feet and two others to lift the trunk. The spine should be kept in line during the manoeuvre. The patient should be moved onto a firm stretcher and one attendant should guard the head and neck during the journey. Oxygen by mask could be given during the ambulance journey.

COURSE

In some patients there may be only a transient paresis. Prognosis may be difficult at first. Spinal shock may last weeks or more.

With a *complete cord lesion*, paralysis and sensory loss do not recover. There is also loss of bowel and bladder control. The affected limbs become spastic, usually in flexion but sometimes in extension. The reflexes are exaggerated and the plantar responses extensor. Muscle spasms may be very troublesome.

IN HOSPITAL

Initially the damage is assessed and examination is made to see if there is any evidence of an unstable spinal fracture. Stable fractures without dislocation are treated by bed rest. Unstable fractures require immobilisation after any dislocation has been reduced. Cervical spine damage may require head traction using Crutchfield tongs applied to the outer skull table. Occasionally internal surgical fixation of an unstable thoraco-lumbar spinal injury is necessary. There is no place for decompressive laminectomies to give the damaged spinal cord 'more room'.

AIMS

To prevent further damage, to allow healing of soft tissue and spinal column injuries, to prevent complications and later to promote an active rehabilitation programme.

NURSING

Regular two hourly turning will prevent pressure sores. Bladder function will be damaged. A few patients, particularly with high cord lesions, may develop an automatic bladder. Most patients require catheterisation – either an in-dwelling catheter or intermittent catheterisation. Infection is always the problem. Later patients may be taught intermittent self-catheterisation eight hourly providing they have sufficiently good hand function. Mild aperients, suppositories, enemata or manual removal will aid defaecation. A bowel action every other day is the aim.

The paralysed limbs are passively exercised daily from the start. As spasticity builds up contractures may develop. Existing active muscles are utilised to their full extent. The aim is for the patient to become independent.

Care of general health is important. 'Silent' urine infections or the development of anaemia may cause ill health with few symptoms and must be excluded.

REHABILITATION

The hospital team consists of doctors, physiotherapists, occupational therapists, appliance fitters, social workers, nurses and even psychologists. These must be supplemented by the patient's family. Work is co-ordinated and intensive. The patient and their relatives should be involved in decision making, e.g. the need to move to a single level accommodation. The patient is instructed in the problems of skin care, bladder control, etc. The outlook must be realistic and outgoing. Morale is maintained by involvement with other paraplegics in social and sporting activities.

Discharge from hospital is a gradual affair with days and weekends at home to begin with. Extensive home adaptations may be necessary and should be organised (and paid for if appropriate) by the Local Authority Social Service Department working with the hospital team. If available, community based occupational therapists, physiotherapists and remedial gymnasts may also help.

Details of the statutory financial support available can be found in the DHSS Office or obtained from the DHSS Leaflet Unit, PO Box 21, Stanmore, Middlesex. A wide range of material covers finance, aids, home adaptations, unemployment, attendance and mobility allowances, holidays, recreation, sex and personal relationships, legislation, contact organisations. Many useful addresses are listed in the Directory for the Disabled (Woodhead Faulkner, 1981).

THE GPs ROLE

About three quarters of the patients who enter spinal centres return 'home'. In the initial few months when the patient is at the spinal centre the main task will be to support the relatives, and if possible visit or make contact with the patient. Most GPs will feel that everyone on the team, and usually the patient, knows a great deal more about the subject than the family doctor. Once the patient returns home, however, the GP will be asked for advice and help. It is important that the family doctor becomes familiar with the objectives that the hospital team have set, and establishes a working relationship with them. It may be necessary to master the technicalities of any apparatus in use and the methods employed in skin care, bladder and bowel function.

Once settled at home the paraplegic is not a great burden on the GP. It is important to supervise bladder function, checking there are no infections. Paraplegics may experience no dysuria or frequency, and may feel no pain even if their skin is ulcerating and underlying bone becoming infected. Such infections occasionally present with an increase in flexor spasms. Prevention of skin damage is the aim.

REFERENCES

1. Fry, J. (1979). *Common Diseases. Their Nature, Incidence and Care*. 2nd Edn. (Lancaster: MTP Press)

2. Hodgkin, K. (1978). *Towards Earlier Diagnosis in Primary Care*. (Edinburgh, London, New York: Churchill Livingstone)

3. Adams, R. D. and Victor, M. (1981). *Principles of Neurology*. 2nd Edn. (USA: McGraw-Hill Company)

4. Lance, J. W. (1969). *The Mechanism and Management of Headache*. (London: Butterworths)

5. Lance, J. W., Curran, D. A. and Anthony, M. (1965). Investigations into the mechanism and treatment of chronic headache. *Med. J. Aust.*, **2**, 909–14

6. Bickerstaff, E. R. (1961). Impairment of consciousness in migraine. *Lancet*, **2**, 1057–9

7. Fowler, T. J. (1980). *Epilepsy*. (London: Update Books Ltd.)

8. Cleland, P. G., Mosquera, I., Steward, W. P. and Foster, J. B. (1981). Prognosis of isolated seizures in adult life. *Br. Med. J.*, **283**, 1364

9. Rutter, N. and Metcalfe, D. H. (1978). Febrile convulsions – what do parents do? *Br. Med. J.*, **2**, 1345–6

10. Stevens, D. L. and Matthews, W.B. (1973). Cryptogenic drop attacks: an affliction of women. *Br. Med. J.*, **1**, 439–42

11. Gowers, W.R. (1885). *Epilepsy and Other Chronic Convulsive Diseases: Their Causes, Symptoms and Treatment*. W. Wood

12. Till, K. (1975). *Paediatric Neurosurgery*. (Oxford, London, Edinburgh, Melbourne: Blackwell Scientific Publications)

13. Gayford, J. J. and Haskell, R. (1979). *Clinical Oral Medicine*. 2nd Edn. (Bristol: J. Wright and Sons Ltd.)

14. Medina, J. L. and Diamond, S. (1981) Cluster headache variant. *Arch. Neurol.*, **38**, 705–9

15. Porter, M. and Jankovic, J. (1981). Benign coital cephalgia. *Arch. Neurol.*, **38**, 710–2

16. Glasspool, M. (1982). *Problems in Ophthalmology*. (Lancaster: MTP Press)

17. Apley, J. (1973). *Paediatrics*. (London: Bailliére Tindall)

18. Geschwind, N. (1972). Language and the brain. *Scientif. Am.*, **226**, 76–83

19. Livesley, B. (1977). The pathogenesis of brain failure in the aged. *Age and Ageing*. (Supplementary Issue Brain Failure in Old Age) *J. Br. Geriatr. Soc.*, 9–13

20. Gilmore, A. J. J. (1974). *Community Surveys and Mental Heath, in Geriatric Medicine*. (London, New York: Academic Press)

21. Kay, D. W. K., Bergmann, K., Foster, E. M., McKechnie, A. A. and Roth, M. (1970) Mental illness and hospital usage in the elderly: a random sample followed up. *Comp. Psychiatry*, **11**, 26–35

22. Hutchinson, E. C., and Acheson, E. J. (1975). *Strokes – Natural History, Pathology and Surgical Treatment*. (London, Philadelphia, Toronto: W. B. Saunders)

23. Fowler, T. J. (1977). *Strokes*. (London: Update Books Ltd.)

24. Sandok, B. A., Furlan, A. J., Whisnant, J. P. and Sundt, T. M. (1978). *Guidelines for the management of TIAs*. Mayo Clin. Proc., **53**, 665–74

25. Fields, W. S., Lemak, N. A., Frankowski, R. F. and Hardy, R. J. (1977). Controlled trial of aspirin in cerebral ischaemia. *Stroke*, **8**, 301–14

26. Teasdale, G. and Jennett, B. (1974). Assessment of coma and impaired consciousness: a practical scale. *Lancet*, **2**, 81–4.

27. Mendelow, A. D., Teasdale, G., Jennett, B., Bryden, J., Hessett, C. and Murray, G. (1983). Risks of intracranial haematoma in head-injured adults. *Br. Med. J.*, **287**, 1173–6

28. Jennett, B. (1975). *Epilepsy after Non-missile Head Injuries*. 2nd Edn. (London: W. Heinemann Medical Books Ltd.)

29. Miller, H. (1961). Accident neurosis. *Br. Med. J.*, 1, 919–25, 992–8

30. Guttmann, L. (1973). *Spinal Cord Injuries*. (Oxford, London, Edinburgh, Melbourne: Blackwell Scientific Publications)

Further reading

Bickerstaff, E. R. (1963). *Neurological Examination in Clinical Practice*. (Oxford: Blackwell Scientific Publications)

Brooke, M. H. (1977). *A Clinician's View of Neuromuscular Diseases*. (Baltimore: Williams and Wilkins)

Cogan, D. G. (1969). *Neurology of the Ocular Muscles*. (Springfield: Charles C. Thomas)

Marshall, J. (1976). *The Management of Cerebrovascular Disease*. (Oxford: Blackwell Scientific Publications)

Matthews, W. B. (1978). *Multiple Sclerosis – The Facts*. (Oxford: Oxford University Press)

Matthews, W. B. and Miller, H. (1972). *Diseases of the Nervous System*. (Oxford, Edinburgh: Blackwell Scientific Publications)

Maurice-Williams, R. S. (1981). *Spinal Degenerative Disease*. (Bristol: J. Wright and Sons Ltd.)

Parkes, J. D. (1982). *Parkinson's Disease*. (London: Update Books Ltd.)

Walton, J. N. (1977). *Brain's Diseases of the Nervous System*. (Oxford: Oxford University Press)

PROPRIETARY DRUG NAMES

Drug Proper Name	Proprietary Name
Amantadine	Symmetrel
Amitriptyline	Lentizol, Tryptizol
Amoxycillin	Amoxil
Baclofen	Lioresal
Benzhexol	Artane
Benztropine	Cogentin
Betahistine	Serc
Bisacodyl	Dulcolax, Dulcodos
Bromocriptine	Parlodel
Carbamazepine	Tegretol
Chloramphenicol	Chlormycetin
Chloroquine	Avloclor, Nivaquine
Chlorpromazine	Largactil
Cinnarizine	Stugeron
Clomipramine	Anafranil
Clonazepam	Rivotril
Clonidine	Dixarit
Dantrolene sodium	Dantrium
Diazepam	Valium, Atensine
Dimenhydrinate	Dramamine
Diphenhydramine	Benadryl
Dothiepin	Prothiaden
Emepronium	Cetiprin
Ethambutol	Myambutol
Ethosuximide	Emeside, Zarontin

Gentamicin	Genticin
Haloperidol	Serenace
Hydralazine	Apresoline
Hydroxocobalamin	Neo-Cytamen
Imipramine	Tofranil
Indomethacin	Indocid
Isoniazid (INAH)	Rimifon
Levodopa	Brocadopa, Larodopa
Levodopa with benserazide	Madopar
Levodopa with carbidopa	Sinemet
Lithium	Camcolit, Priadel
Lorazepam	Almazine, Ativan
Methylphenidate	Ritalin
Methysergide	Deseril
Metoclopramide	Maxolon
Metrizamide	Amipaque
Metronidazole	Flagyl, Metrolyl, Zadstat
Naproxen sodium	Naprosyn, Synflex
Neostigmine	Prostigmin
Nitrazepam	Mogadon
Nitrofurantoin	Berkfurin, Furadantin, Macrodantin
Nomifensine	Merital
Orphenadrine	Disipal
Paracetamol	Panadol, Calpol
Penicillamine	Distamine

206

Perphenazine	Fentazin
Phenobarbitone	Gardenal, Luminal
Phenytoin	Epanutin, Dilantin
Pimozide	Orap
Pizotifen	Sanomigran
Prednisolone	Deltacortril, Deltastab, Prednesol
Primidone	Mysoline
Prochlorperazine	Stemetil, Vertigon
Promethazine	Phenergan
Propantheline	Pro-Banthine
Propranolol	Berkolol, Inderal
Pyridostigmine	Mestinon
Selegiline	Eldepryl
Sodium valproate	Epilim
Sterculia	Normacol
Tetrabenazine	Nitoman
Thiopropazate	Dartalan
Thioridazine	Melleril
Trimipramine	Surmontil
Tropicamide	Mydriacyl
Valproate sodium	Epilim
Vincristine	Oncovin

Index

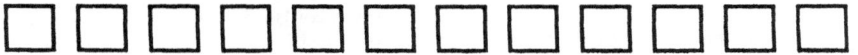

215